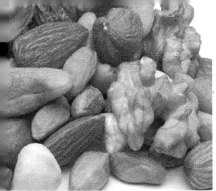
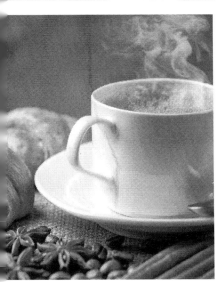
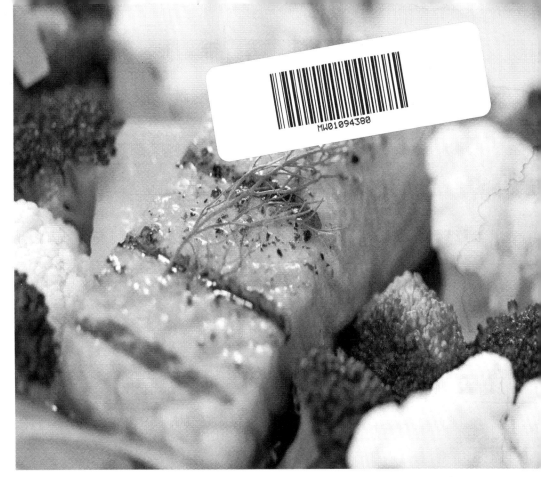

Acid Reflux & GERD
60-Day Food Journal

Detailed recording log to identify problem foods, drinks, meds, and habits.

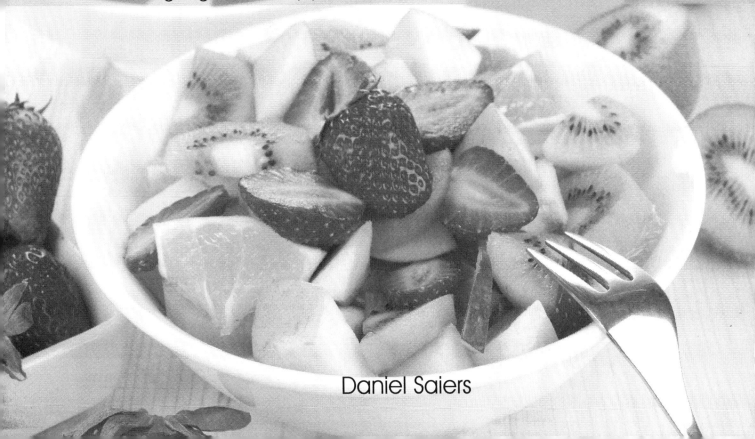

Daniel Saiers

MW01094380

DATE

Breakfast   Time: _____

List the foods you ate for breakfast.

_____   _____

_____   _____

_____   _____

Drink _____   **Drink** _____
○ room-temp ○ hot ○ cold   ○ room-temp ○ hot ○ cold

Comments:

Physical symptoms after meal: ○ **low**   ○ **intense**   ○ **non-existent**
○ Belching   ○ Upper abdominal pain and discomfort
○ Nausea   ○ Difficulty or pain with swallowing
○ Stomach fullness or bloating   ○ Wheezing or dry cough

Other symptoms:

Post-breakfast energy level: ○ low ○ medium ○ high

Lunch   Time: _____

List the foods you ate for lunch.

_____   _____

_____   _____

_____   _____

Drink _____   **Drink** _____
○ room-temp ○ hot ○ cold   ○ room-temp ○ hot ○ cold

Comments:

Physical symptoms after meal: ○ **low**   ○ **intense**   ○ **non-existent**
○ Belching   ○ Upper abdominal pain and discomfort
○ Nausea   ○ Difficulty or pain with swallowing
○ Stomach fullness or bloating   ○ Wheezing or dry cough

Other symptoms:

Post-lunch energy level: ○ low ○ medium ○ high

Dinner

Time: _____

List the foods you ate for dinner.

_____   _____

_____   _____

_____   _____

Drink _____   **Drink** _____
○ room-temp ○ hot ○ cold   ○ room-temp ○ hot ○ cold

Comments: _____

Physical symptoms after meal: ○ **low** ○ **intense** ○ **non-existent**
○ Belching   ○ Upper abdominal pain and discomfort
○ Nausea   ○ Difficulty or pain with swallowing
○ Stomach fullness or bloating ○ Wheezing or dry cough

Other symptoms: _____

Post-dinner energy level: ○ low ○ medium ○ high

Snack

Time: _____

List the foods you ate as a snack.

_____   _____

Drink _____   ○ room-temp ○ hot ○ cold

Comments: _____

Post-snack energy level: ○ low ○ medium ○ high

Snack

Time: _____

List the foods you ate as a snack.

_____   _____

Drink _____   ○ room-temp ○ hot ○ cold

Comments: _____

Post-snack energy level: ○ low ○ medium ○ high

Medications & Supplements

Include prescription medication, over-the-counter medication & vitamin supplements.

_____   _____

_____   _____

_____   _____

_____   _____

_____   _____

Energy level | Restfulness

Today's waking energy level?
○ low   ○ medium   ○ high

# of times roused from sleep last night?
○ 1   ○ 2   ○ 3+

Last night's reflux/GERD symptoms:

_____   _____

_____   _____

Bed raised?   ○ Y   ○ N   Wedged Pillows?   ○ Y   ○ N

Last meal time? _____   Approx bedtime? _____ am pm

(Remember to give yourself at least 2-3 hours after meals before lying down.)

End-of-day notes

Noticeable change in symptoms? *(Ex: "Throat discomfort has completely disappeared.")*

_____

_____

New terms to research   Books & websites with helpful info

_____   _____

_____   _____

Additional notes:

_____

_____

_____

Breakfast   Time: _____

List the foods you ate for breakfast.

_____   _____

_____   _____

_____   _____

Drink _____   **Drink** _____
○ room-temp   ○ hot   ○ cold   ○ room-temp   ○ hot   ○ cold

Comments: _____

Physical symptoms after meal: ○ **low**   ○ **intense**   ○ **non-existent**
○ Belching   ○ Upper abdominal pain and discomfort
○ Nausea   ○ Difficulty or pain with swallowing
○ Stomach fullness or bloating   ○ Wheezing or dry cough

Other symptoms: _____

Post-breakfast energy level: ○ low   ○ medium   ○ high

Lunch   Time: _____

List the foods you ate for lunch.

_____   _____

_____   _____

_____   _____

Drink _____   **Drink** _____
○ room-temp   ○ hot   ○ cold   ○ room-temp   ○ hot   ○ cold

Comments: _____

Physical symptoms after meal: ○ **low**   ○ **intense**   ○ **non-existent**
○ Belching   ○ Upper abdominal pain and discomfort
○ Nausea   ○ Difficulty or pain with swallowing
○ Stomach fullness or bloating   ○ Wheezing or dry cough

Other symptoms: _____

Post-lunch energy level: ○ low   ○ medium   ○ high

Dinner

Time: _____

List the foods you ate for dinner.

_____   _____

_____   _____

_____   _____

Drink _____   **Drink** _____
○ room-temp ○ hot ○ cold   ○ room-temp ○ hot ○ cold

Comments: _____

Physical symptoms after meal: ○ **low**   ○ **intense**   ○ **non-existent**
○ Belching   ○ Upper abdominal pain and discomfort
○ Nausea   ○ Difficulty or pain with swallowing
○ Stomach fullness or bloating   ○ Wheezing or dry cough

Other symptoms: _____

Post-dinner energy level: ○ low   ○ medium   ○ high

Snack

Time: _____

List the foods you ate as a snack.

_____   _____

Drink _____   ○ room-temp   ○ hot   ○ cold

Comments: _____

Post-snack energy level: ○ low   ○ medium   ○ high

Snack

Time: _____

List the foods you ate as a snack.

_____   _____

Drink _____   ○ room-temp   ○ hot   ○ cold

Comments: _____

Post-snack energy level: ○ low   ○ medium   ○ high

Medications & Supplements

Include prescription medication, over-the-counter medication & vitamin supplements.

_____   _____

_____   _____

_____   _____

_____   _____

_____   _____

Energy level | Restfulness

Today's waking energy level?
○ low   ○ medium   ○ high

# of times roused from sleep last night?
○ 1   ○ 2   ○ 3+

Last night's reflux/GERD symptoms:

_____   _____

_____   _____

Bed raised?   ○ Y   ○ N   Wedged Pillows?   ○ Y   ○ N

Last meal time? _____   Approx bedtime? _____ am pm
(Remember to give yourself at least 2-3 hours after meals before lying down.)

End-of-day notes

Noticeable change in symptoms? _(Ex: "Throat discomfort has completely disappeared.")_

_____

_____

New terms to research   Books & websites with helpful info

_____   _____

_____   _____

Additional notes:

_____

_____

_____

Breakfast
Time: _____

List the foods you ate for breakfast.

_____   _____

_____   _____

_____   _____

Drink _____   **Drink** _____
○ room-temp ○ hot ○ cold   ○ room-temp ○ hot ○ cold

Comments:

Physical symptoms after meal: ○ **low** ○ **intense** ○ **non-existent**
○ Belching   ○ Upper abdominal pain and discomfort
○ Nausea   ○ Difficulty or pain with swallowing
○ Stomach fullness or bloating   ○ Wheezing or dry cough

Other symptoms:

Post-breakfast energy level: ○ low ○ medium ○ high

Lunch
Time: _____

List the foods you ate for lunch.

_____   _____

_____   _____

_____   _____

Drink _____   **Drink** _____
○ room-temp ○ hot ○ cold   ○ room-temp ○ hot ○ cold

Comments:

Physical symptoms after meal: ○ **low** ○ **intense** ○ **non-existent**
○ Belching   ○ Upper abdominal pain and discomfort
○ Nausea   ○ Difficulty or pain with swallowing
○ Stomach fullness or bloating   ○ Wheezing or dry cough

Other symptoms:

Post-lunch energy level: ○ low ○ medium ○ high

Dinner

Time: _____

List the foods you ate for dinner.

_____   _____

_____   _____

_____   _____

Drink _____   **Drink** _____
○ room-temp ○ hot ○ cold   ○ room-temp ○ hot ○ cold

Comments:

Physical symptoms after meal: ○ **low** ○ **intense** ○ **non-existent**
○ Belching   ○ Upper abdominal pain and discomfort
○ Nausea   ○ Difficulty or pain with swallowing
○ Stomach fullness or bloating   ○ Wheezing or dry cough

Other symptoms:

Post-dinner energy level: ○ low ○ medium ○ high

Snack

Time: _____

List the foods you ate as a snack.

_____   _____

Drink _____   ○ room-temp ○ hot ○ cold

Comments:

Post-snack energy level: ○ low ○ medium ○ high

Snack

Time: _____

List the foods you ate as a snack.

_____   _____

Drink _____   ○ room-temp ○ hot ○ cold

Comments:

Post-snack energy level: ○ low ○ medium ○ high

Medications & Supplements
Include prescription medication, over-the-counter medication & vitamin supplements.

_____   _____

_____   _____

_____   _____

_____   _____

_____   _____

Energy level | Restfulness

Today's waking energy level?
○ low   ○ medium   ○ high

# of times roused from sleep last night?
○ 1   ○ 2   ○ 3+

Last night's reflux/GERD symptoms:

_____   _____

_____   _____

Bed raised?   ○ Y   ○ N   Wedged Pillows?   ○ Y   ○ N

Last meal time? _____   Approx bedtime? _____ am pm
(Remember to give yourself at least 2-3 hours after meals before lying down.)

End-of-day notes

Noticeable change in symptoms? _(Ex: "Throat discomfort has completely disappeared.")_

_____

_____

New terms to research   Books & websites with helpful info

_____   _____

_____   _____

Additional notes:

_____

_____

_____

Breakfast

Time: _____

List the foods you ate for breakfast.

_____   _____

_____   _____

_____   _____

Drink _____   **Drink** _____
○ room-temp   ○ hot   ○ cold   ○ room-temp   ○ hot   ○ cold

_____

Physical symptoms after meal: ○ **low**   ○ **intense**   ○ **non-existent**
○ Belching   ○ Upper abdominal pain and discomfort
○ Nausea   ○ Difficulty or pain with swallowing
○ Stomach fullness or bloating   ○ Wheezing or dry cough

Other symptoms: _____

Post-breakfast energy level: ○ low   ○ medium   ○ high

Lunch

Time: _____

List the foods you ate for lunch.

_____   _____

_____   _____

_____   _____

Drink _____   **Drink** _____
○ room-temp   ○ hot   ○ cold   ○ room-temp   ○ hot   ○ cold

Comments:
_____

Physical symptoms after meal: ○ **low**   ○ **intense**   ○ **non-existent**
○ Belching   ○ Upper abdominal pain and discomfort
○ Nausea   ○ Difficulty or pain with swallowing
○ Stomach fullness or bloating   ○ Wheezing or dry cough

Other symptoms: _____

Post-lunch energy level: ○ low   ○ medium   ○ high

Dinner

Time: _____

List the foods you ate for dinner.

_____   _____

_____   _____

_____   _____

Drink _____   **Drink** _____
○ room-temp   ○ hot   ○ cold   ○ room-temp   ○ hot   ○ cold

Comments:

_____

Physical symptoms after meal: ○ **low**   ○ **intense**   ○ **non-existent**
○ Belching   ○ Upper abdominal pain and discomfort
○ Nausea   ○ Difficulty or pain with swallowing
○ Stomach fullness or bloating   ○ Wheezing or dry cough

Other symptoms:

_____

Post-dinner energy level: ○ low   ○ medium   ○ high

Snack

Time: _____

List the foods you ate as a snack.

_____   _____

Drink _____   ○ room-temp   ○ hot   ○ cold

Comments: _____

Post-snack energy level: ○ low   ○ medium   ○ high

Snack

Time: _____

List the foods you ate as a snack.

_____   _____

Drink _____   ○ room-temp   ○ hot   ○ cold

Comments: _____

Post-snack energy level: ○ low   ○ medium   ○ high

Medications & Supplements

Include prescription medication, over-the-counter medication & vitamin supplements.

_____   _____

_____   _____

_____   _____

_____   _____

_____   _____

Energy level | Restfulness

Today's waking energy level?
○ low   ○ medium   ○ high

# of times roused from sleep last night?
○ 1   ○ 2   ○ 3+

Last night's reflux/GERD symptoms:

_____   _____

_____   _____

Bed raised?   ○ Y   ○ N   Wedged Pillows?   ○ Y   ○ N

Last meal time? _____   Approx bedtime? _____   am   pm
(Remember to give yourself at least 2-3 hours after meals before lying down.)

End-of-day notes

Noticeable change in symptoms? _(Ex: "Throat discomfort has completely disappeared.")_

_____

_____

New terms to research   Books & websites with helpful info

_____   _____

_____   _____

Additional notes:

_____

_____

_____

Breakfast   Time: _____

List the foods you ate for breakfast.

_____   _____

_____   _____

_____   _____

Drink _____   **Drink** _____
○ room-temp   ○ hot   ○ cold   ○ room-temp   ○ hot   ○ cold

Comments:

Physical symptoms after meal: ○ **low**   ○ **intense**   ○ **non-existent**
○ Belching   ○ Upper abdominal pain and discomfort
○ Nausea   ○ Difficulty or pain with swallowing
○ Stomach fullness or bloating   ○ Wheezing or dry cough

Other symptoms:

Post-breakfast energy level: ○ low   ○ medium   ○ high

Lunch   Time: _____

List the foods you ate for lunch.

_____   _____

_____   _____

_____   _____

Drink _____   **Drink** _____
○ room-temp   ○ hot   ○ cold   ○ room-temp   ○ hot   ○ cold

Comments:

Physical symptoms after meal: ○ **low**   ○ **intense**   ○ **non-existent**
○ Belching   ○ Upper abdominal pain and discomfort
○ Nausea   ○ Difficulty or pain with swallowing
○ Stomach fullness or bloating   ○ Wheezing or dry cough

Other symptoms:

Post-lunch energy level: ○ low   ○ medium   ○ high

Dinner

Time: _____

List the foods you ate for dinner.

_____   _____

_____   _____

_____   _____

Drink _____   **Drink** _____
    ○ room-temp   ○ hot   ○ cold   ○ room-temp   ○ hot   ○ cold

Comments: _____

Physical symptoms after meal: ○ **low**   ○ **intense**   ○ **non-existent**

○ Belching   ○ Upper abdominal pain and discomfort

○ Nausea   ○ Difficulty or pain with swallowing

○ Stomach fullness or bloating   ○ Wheezing or dry cough

Other symptoms: _____

Post-dinner energy level: ○ low   ○ medium   ○ high

Snack

Time: _____

List the foods you ate as a snack.

_____   _____

Drink _____   ○ room-temp   ○ hot   ○ cold

Comments: _____

Post-snack energy level: ○ low   ○ medium   ○ high

Snack

Time: _____

List the foods you ate as a snack.

_____   _____

Drink _____   ○ room-temp   ○ hot   ○ cold

Comments: _____

Post-snack energy level: ○ low   ○ medium   ○ high

Medications & Supplements

Include prescription medication, over-the-counter medication & vitamin supplements.

_____   _____

_____   _____

_____   _____

_____   _____

_____   _____

Energy level | Restfulness

Today's waking energy level?
○ low   ○ medium   ○ high

# of times roused from sleep last night?
○ 1   ○ 2   ○ 3+

Last night's reflux/GERD symptoms:

_____   _____

_____   _____

Bed raised?   ○ Y   ○ N   Wedged Pillows?   ○ Y   ○ N

Last meal time? _____   Approx bedtime? _____ am pm
(Remember to give yourself at least 2-3 hours after meals before lying down.)

End-of-day notes

Noticeable change in symptoms? _(Ex: "Throat discomfort has completely disappeared.")_

_____

_____

New terms to research   Books & websites with helpful info

_____   _____

_____   _____

Additional notes:

_____

_____

_____

Breakfast   Time: _____

List the foods you ate for breakfast.

_____   _____

_____   _____

_____   _____

🥤 **Drink** _____   **Drink** _____
  ○ room-temp ○ hot ○ cold   ○ room-temp ○ hot ○ cold

Comments: _____

Physical symptoms after meal: ○ **low** ○ **intense** ○ **non-existent**
○ Belching   ○ Upper abdominal pain and discomfort
○ Nausea   ○ Difficulty or pain with swallowing
○ Stomach fullness or bloating   ○ Wheezing or dry cough

Other symptoms: _____

Post-breakfast energy level: ○ low   ○ medium   ○ high

Lunch   Time: _____

List the foods you ate for lunch.

_____   _____

_____   _____

_____   _____

🥤 **Drink** _____   **Drink** _____
  ○ room-temp ○ hot ○ cold   ○ room-temp ○ hot ○ cold

Comments: _____

Physical symptoms after meal: ○ **low** ○ **intense** ○ **non-existent**
○ Belching   ○ Upper abdominal pain and discomfort
○ Nausea   ○ Difficulty or pain with swallowing
○ Stomach fullness or bloating   ○ Wheezing or dry cough

Other symptoms: _____

Post-lunch energy level: ○ low   ○ medium   ○ high

Dinner

Time: _____

List the foods you ate for dinner.

_____   _____

_____   _____

_____   _____

Drink _____   **Drink** _____
○ room-temp   ○ hot   ○ cold   ○ room-temp   ○ hot   ○ cold

Comments: _____

Physical symptoms after meal: ○ **low**   ○ **intense**   ○ **non-existent**
○ Belching   ○ Upper abdominal pain and discomfort
○ Nausea   ○ Difficulty or pain with swallowing
○ Stomach fullness or bloating   ○ Wheezing or dry cough

Other symptoms: _____

Post-dinner energy level: ○ low   ○ medium   ○ high

Snack

Time: _____

List the foods you ate as a snack.

_____   _____

Drink _____   ○ room-temp   ○ hot   ○ cold

Comments: _____

Post-snack energy level: ○ low   ○ medium   ○ high

Snack

Time: _____

List the foods you ate as a snack.

_____   _____

Drink _____   ○ room-temp   ○ hot   ○ cold

Comments: _____

Post-snack energy level: ○ low   ○ medium   ○ high

Medications & Supplements

Include prescription medication, over-the-counter medication & vitamin supplements.

_____   _____

_____   _____

_____   _____

_____   _____

_____   _____

Energy level | Restfulness

Today's waking energy level?
○ low   ○ medium   ○ high

# of times roused from sleep last night?
○ 1   ○ 2   ○ 3+

Last night's reflux/GERD symptoms:

_____   _____

_____   _____

Bed raised?   ○ Y   ○ N   Wedged Pillows?   ○ Y   ○ N

Last meal time? _____   Approx bedtime? _____   am   pm
(Remember to give yourself at least 2-3 hours after meals before lying down.)

End-of-day notes

Noticeable change in symptoms? *(Ex: "Throat discomfort has completely disappeared.")*

_____

_____

New terms to research   Books & websites with helpful info

_____   _____

_____   _____

Additional notes:

_____

_____

_____

Breakfast   Time: _____

List the foods you ate for breakfast.

_____   _____

_____   _____

_____   _____

Drink _____   **Drink** _____
○ room-temp   ○ hot   ○ cold   ○ room-temp   ○ hot   ○ cold

Comments:

Physical symptoms after meal: ○ **low**   ○ **intense**   ○ **non-existent**
○ Belching   ○ Upper abdominal pain and discomfort
○ Nausea   ○ Difficulty or pain with swallowing
○ Stomach fullness or bloating   ○ Wheezing or dry cough

Other symptoms:

Post-breakfast energy level: ○ low   ○ medium   ○ high

Lunch   Time: _____

List the foods you ate for lunch.

_____   _____

_____   _____

_____   _____

Drink _____   **Drink** _____
○ room-temp   ○ hot   ○ cold   ○ room-temp   ○ hot   ○ cold

Comments:

Physical symptoms after meal: ○ **low**   ○ **intense**   ○ **non-existent**
○ Belching   ○ Upper abdominal pain and discomfort
○ Nausea   ○ Difficulty or pain with swallowing
○ Stomach fullness or bloating   ○ Wheezing or dry cough

Other symptoms:

Post-lunch energy level: ○ low   ○ medium   ○ high

Dinner

Time: _____

List the foods you ate for dinner.

_____   _____

_____   _____

_____   _____

Drink _____   **Drink** _____
○ room-temp   ○ hot   ○ cold   ○ room-temp   ○ hot   ○ cold

Comments: _____

Physical symptoms after meal: ○ **low**   ○ **intense**   ○ **non-existent**
○ Belching   ○ Upper abdominal pain and discomfort
○ Nausea   ○ Difficulty or pain with swallowing
○ Stomach fullness or bloating   ○ Wheezing or dry cough

Other symptoms: _____

Post-dinner energy level: ○ low   ○ medium   ○ high

Snack

Time: _____

List the foods you ate as a snack.

_____   _____

Drink _____   ○ room-temp   ○ hot   ○ cold

Comments: _____

Post-snack energy level: ○ low   ○ medium   ○ high

Snack

Time: _____

List the foods you ate as a snack.

_____   _____

Drink _____   ○ room-temp   ○ hot   ○ cold

Comments: _____

Post-snack energy level: ○ low   ○ medium   ○ high

Medications & Supplements

Include prescription medication, over-the-counter medication & vitamin supplements.

_____   _____

_____   _____

_____   _____

_____   _____

_____   _____

Energy level | Restfulness

Today's waking energy level?
○ low   ○ medium   ○ high

# of times roused from sleep last night?
○ 1   ○ 2   ○ 3+

Last night's reflux/GERD symptoms:

_____   _____

_____   _____

Bed raised?   ○ Y   ○ N   Wedged Pillows?   ○ Y   ○ N

Last meal time? _____   Approx bedtime? _____   am   pm
(Remember to give yourself at least 2-3 hours after meals before lying down.)

End-of-day notes

Noticeable change in symptoms? *(Ex: "Throat discomfort has completely disappeared.")*

_____

_____

New terms to research   Books & websites with helpful info

_____   _____

_____   _____

Additional notes:

_____

_____

_____

Breakfast   Time: _____

List the foods you ate for breakfast.

_____   _____

_____   _____

_____   _____

Drink _____   **Drink** _____
○ room-temp ○ hot ○ cold   ○ room-temp ○ hot ○ cold

Comments: _____

Physical symptoms after meal: ○ **low**   ○ **intense**   ○ **non-existent**
○ Belching   ○ Upper abdominal pain and discomfort
○ Nausea   ○ Difficulty or pain with swallowing
○ Stomach fullness or bloating   ○ Wheezing or dry cough

Other symptoms: _____

Post-breakfast energy level: ○ low ○ medium ○ high

Lunch   Time: _____

List the foods you ate for lunch.

_____   _____

_____   _____

_____   _____

Drink _____   **Drink** _____
○ room-temp ○ hot ○ cold   ○ room-temp ○ hot ○ cold

Comments: _____

Physical symptoms after meal: ○ **low**   ○ **intense**   ○ **non-existent**
○ Belching   ○ Upper abdominal pain and discomfort
○ Nausea   ○ Difficulty or pain with swallowing
○ Stomach fullness or bloating   ○ Wheezing or dry cough

Other symptoms: _____

Post-lunch energy level: ○ low ○ medium ○ high

Dinner

Time: _____

List the foods you ate for dinner.

_____   _____

_____   _____

_____   _____

Drink _____   **Drink** _____
○ room-temp ○ hot ○ cold   ○ room-temp ○ hot ○ cold

Comments:
_____

Physical symptoms after meal: ○ **low** ○ **intense** ○ **non-existent**
○ Belching   ○ Upper abdominal pain and discomfort
○ Nausea   ○ Difficulty or pain with swallowing
○ Stomach fullness or bloating ○ Wheezing or dry cough

Other symptoms:
_____

Post-dinner energy level: ○ low ○ medium ○ high

Snack

Time: _____

List the foods you ate as a snack.

_____   _____

Drink _____   ○ room-temp ○ hot ○ cold

Comments:
_____

Post-snack energy level: ○ low ○ medium ○ high

Snack

Time: _____

List the foods you ate as a snack.

_____   _____

Drink _____   ○ room-temp ○ hot ○ cold

Comments:
_____

Post-snack energy level: ○ low ○ medium ○ high

Medications & Supplements

Include prescription medication, over-the-counter medication & vitamin supplements.

_____   _____

_____   _____

_____   _____

_____   _____

Energy level | Restfulness

Today's waking energy level?
○ low   ○ medium   ○ high

# of times roused from sleep last night?
○ 1   ○ 2   ○ 3+

Last night's reflux/GERD symptoms:

_____   _____

_____   _____

Bed raised?   ○ Y   ○ N   Wedged Pillows?   ○ Y   ○ N

Last meal time? _____   Approx bedtime? _____   am   pm
(Remember to give yourself at least 2-3 hours after meals before lying down.)

End-of-day notes

Noticeable change in symptoms? _(Ex: "Throat discomfort has completely disappeared.")_

_____

_____

New terms to research   Books & websites with helpful info

_____   _____

_____   _____

Additional notes:

_____

_____

_____

Breakfast

Time: _____

List the foods you ate for breakfast.

_____   _____

_____   _____

_____   _____

Drink _____   **Drink** _____
○ room-temp ○ hot ○ cold   ○ room-temp ○ hot ○ cold

Comments:

Physical symptoms after meal: ○ **low**   ○ **intense**   ○ **non-existent**
○ Belching   ○ Upper abdominal pain and discomfort
○ Nausea   ○ Difficulty or pain with swallowing
○ Stomach fullness or bloating   ○ Wheezing or dry cough

Other symptoms:

Post-breakfast energy level: ○ low   ○ medium   ○ high

Lunch

Time: _____

List the foods you ate for lunch.

_____   _____

_____   _____

_____   _____

Drink _____   **Drink** _____
○ room-temp ○ hot ○ cold   ○ room-temp ○ hot ○ cold

Comments:

Physical symptoms after meal: ○ **low**   ○ **intense**   ○ **non-existent**
○ Belching   ○ Upper abdominal pain and discomfort
○ Nausea   ○ Difficulty or pain with swallowing
○ Stomach fullness or bloating   ○ Wheezing or dry cough

Other symptoms:

Post-lunch energy level: ○ low   ○ medium   ○ high

Dinner

Time: _____

List the foods you ate for dinner.

_____   _____

_____   _____

_____   _____

Drink _____   **Drink** _____
○ room-temp ○ hot ○ cold   ○ room-temp ○ hot ○ cold

Comments: _____

Physical symptoms after meal: ○ **low**   ○ **intense**   ○ **non-existent**
○ Belching   ○ Upper abdominal pain and discomfort
○ Nausea   ○ Difficulty or pain with swallowing
○ Stomach fullness or bloating   ○ Wheezing or dry cough

Other symptoms: _____

Post-dinner energy level: ○ low   ○ medium   ○ high

Snack

Time: _____

List the foods you ate as a snack.

_____   _____

Drink _____   ○ room-temp   ○ hot   ○ cold

Comments: _____

Post-snack energy level: ○ low   ○ medium   ○ high

Snack

Time: _____

List the foods you ate as a snack.

_____   _____

Drink _____   ○ room-temp   ○ hot   ○ cold

Comments: _____

Post-snack energy level: ○ low   ○ medium   ○ high

Medications & Supplements

Include prescription medication, over-the-counter medication & vitamin supplements.

_____   _____

_____   _____

_____   _____

_____   _____

_____   _____

Energy level | Restfulness

Today's waking energy level?
○ low   ○ medium   ○ high

# of times roused from sleep last night?
○ 1   ○ 2   ○ 3+

Last night's reflux/GERD symptoms:

_____   _____

_____   _____

Bed raised?   ○ Y   ○ N   Wedged Pillows?   ○ Y   ○ N

Last meal time? _____   Approx bedtime? _____ am pm
        (Remember to give yourself at least 2-3 hours after meals before lying down.)

End-of-day notes

Noticeable change in symptoms? _(Ex: "Throat discomfort has completely disappeared.")_

_____

_____

New terms to research   Books & websites with helpful info

_____   _____

_____   _____

Additional notes:

_____

_____

_____

Breakfast   Time: _____

List the foods you ate for breakfast.

_____   _____

_____   _____

_____   _____

Drink _____   **Drink** _____
○ room-temp ○ hot ○ cold   ○ room-temp ○ hot ○ cold

Comments: _____

Physical symptoms after meal: ○ **low**   ○ **intense**   ○ **non-existent**
○ Belching   ○ Upper abdominal pain and discomfort
○ Nausea   ○ Difficulty or pain with swallowing
○ Stomach fullness or bloating   ○ Wheezing or dry cough

Other symptoms: _____

Post-breakfast energy level: ○ low   ○ medium   ○ high

Lunch   Time: _____

List the foods you ate for lunch.

_____   _____

_____   _____

_____   _____

Drink _____   **Drink** _____
○ room-temp ○ hot ○ cold   ○ room-temp ○ hot ○ cold

Comments: _____

Physical symptoms after meal: ○ **low**   ○ **intense**   ○ **non-existent**
○ Belching   ○ Upper abdominal pain and discomfort
○ Nausea   ○ Difficulty or pain with swallowing
○ Stomach fullness or bloating   ○ Wheezing or dry cough

Other symptoms: _____

Post-lunch energy level: ○ low   ○ medium   ○ high

Dinner

Time: _____

List the foods you ate for dinner.

_____   _____

_____   _____

_____   _____

Drink _____   **Drink** _____
○ room-temp   ○ hot   ○ cold   ○ room-temp   ○ hot   ○ cold

Comments: _____

Physical symptoms after meal: ○ **low**   ○ **intense**   ○ **non-existent**
○ Belching   ○ Upper abdominal pain and discomfort
○ Nausea   ○ Difficulty or pain with swallowing
○ Stomach fullness or bloating   ○ Wheezing or dry cough

Other symptoms: _____

Post-dinner energy level: ○ low   ○ medium   ○ high

Snack

Time: _____

List the foods you ate as a snack.

_____   _____

Drink _____   ○ room-temp   ○ hot   ○ cold

Comments: _____

Post-snack energy level: ○ low   ○ medium   ○ high

Snack

Time: _____

List the foods you ate as a snack.

_____   _____

Drink _____   ○ room-temp   ○ hot   ○ cold

Comments: _____

Post-snack energy level: ○ low   ○ medium   ○ high

Medications & Supplements

Include prescription medication, over-the-counter medication & vitamin supplements.

_____   _____

_____   _____

_____   _____

_____   _____

_____   _____

Energy level | Restfulness

Today's waking energy level?
○ low   ○ medium   ○ high

# of times roused from sleep last night?
○ 1   ○ 2   ○ 3+

Last night's reflux/GERD symptoms:

_____   _____

_____   _____

Bed raised?   ○ Y   ○ N   Wedged Pillows?   ○ Y   ○ N

Last meal time? _____   Approx bedtime? _____   am   pm
(Remember to give yourself at least 2-3 hours after meals before lying down.)

End-of-day notes

Noticeable change in symptoms? *(Ex: "Throat discomfort has completely disappeared.")*

_____

_____

New terms to research   Books & websites with helpful info

_____   _____

_____   _____

Additional notes:

_____

_____

_____

Breakfast
Time: _____

List the foods you ate for breakfast.

_____   _____

_____   _____

_____   _____

Drink _____   **Drink** _____
○ room-temp ○ hot ○ cold   ○ room-temp ○ hot ○ cold

Comments:

Physical symptoms after meal: ○ **low**   ○ **intense**   ○ **non-existent**
○ Belching   ○ Upper abdominal pain and discomfort
○ Nausea   ○ Difficulty or pain with swallowing
○ Stomach fullness or bloating   ○ Wheezing or dry cough

Other symptoms:

Post-breakfast energy level: ○ low ○ medium ○ high

Lunch
Time: _____

List the foods you ate for lunch.

_____   _____

_____   _____

_____   _____

Drink _____   **Drink** _____
○ room-temp ○ hot ○ cold   ○ room-temp ○ hot ○ cold

Comments:

Physical symptoms after meal: ○ **low**   ○ **intense**   ○ **non-existent**
○ Belching   ○ Upper abdominal pain and discomfort
○ Nausea   ○ Difficulty or pain with swallowing
○ Stomach fullness or bloating   ○ Wheezing or dry cough

Other symptoms:

Post-lunch energy level: ○ low ○ medium ○ high

Dinner   Time: _____

List the foods you ate for dinner.

_____   _____

_____   _____

_____   _____

Drink _____   **Drink** _____
  ○ room-temp ○ hot ○ cold   ○ room-temp ○ hot ○ cold

Comments: _____

Physical symptoms after meal: ○ **low**   ○ **intense**   ○ **non-existent**
○ Belching   ○ Upper abdominal pain and discomfort
○ Nausea   ○ Difficulty or pain with swallowing
○ Stomach fullness or bloating   ○ Wheezing or dry cough

Other symptoms: _____

Post-dinner energy level: ○ low   ○ medium   ○ high

Snack   Time: _____

List the foods you ate as a snack.

_____   _____

Drink _____   ○ room-temp   ○ hot   ○ cold

Comments: _____

Post-snack energy level: ○ low   ○ medium   ○ high

Snack   Time: _____

List the foods you ate as a snack.

_____   _____

Drink _____   ○ room-temp   ○ hot   ○ cold

Comments: _____

Post-snack energy level: ○ low   ○ medium   ○ high

Medications & Supplements

Include prescription medication, over-the-counter medication & vitamin supplements.

_____   _____

_____   _____

_____   _____

_____   _____

_____   _____

Energy level | Restfulness

Today's waking energy level?
○ low   ○ medium   ○ high

# of times roused from sleep last night?
○ 1   ○ 2   ○ 3+

Last night's reflux/GERD symptoms:

_____   _____

_____   _____

Bed raised?   ○ Y   ○ N   Wedged Pillows?   ○ Y   ○ N

Last meal time? _____   Approx bedtime? _____ am pm

(Remember to give yourself at least 2-3 hours after meals before lying down.)

End-of-day notes

Noticeable change in symptoms? *(Ex: "Throat discomfort has completely disappeared.")*

_____

_____

New terms to research   Books & websites with helpful info

_____   _____

_____   _____

Additional notes:

_____

_____

_____

_____

Breakfast   Time: _____

List the foods you ate for breakfast.

_____   _____

_____   _____

_____   _____

Drink _____   **Drink** _____
○ room-temp   ○ hot   ○ cold   ○ room-temp   ○ hot   ○ cold

Comments: _____

Physical symptoms after meal: ○ **low**   ○ **intense**   ○ **non-existent**
○ Belching   ○ Upper abdominal pain and discomfort
○ Nausea   ○ Difficulty or pain with swallowing
○ Stomach fullness or bloating   ○ Wheezing or dry cough

Other symptoms: _____

Post-breakfast energy level: ○ low   ○ medium   ○ high

Lunch   Time: _____

List the foods you ate for lunch.

_____   _____

_____   _____

_____   _____

Drink _____   **Drink** _____
○ room-temp   ○ hot   ○ cold   ○ room-temp   ○ hot   ○ cold

Comments: _____

Physical symptoms after meal: ○ **low**   ○ **intense**   ○ **non-existent**
○ Belching   ○ Upper abdominal pain and discomfort
○ Nausea   ○ Difficulty or pain with swallowing
○ Stomach fullness or bloating   ○ Wheezing or dry cough

Other symptoms: _____

Post-lunch energy level: ○ low   ○ medium   ○ high

Dinner

Time: _____

List the foods you ate for dinner.

_____   _____

_____   _____

_____   _____

Drink _____   **Drink** _____
○ room-temp   ○ hot   ○ cold   ○ room-temp   ○ hot   ○ cold

Comments:
_____

Physical symptoms after meal: ○ **low**   ○ **intense**   ○ **non-existent**
○ Belching   ○ Upper abdominal pain and discomfort
○ Nausea   ○ Difficulty or pain with swallowing
○ Stomach fullness or bloating   ○ Wheezing or dry cough

Other symptoms:

Post-dinner energy level: ○ low   ○ medium   ○ high

Snack

Time: _____

List the foods you ate as a snack.

_____   _____

Drink _____   ○ room-temp   ○ hot   ○ cold

Comments: _____

Post-snack energy level: ○ low   ○ medium   ○ high

Snack

Time: _____

List the foods you ate as a snack.

_____   _____

Drink _____   ○ room-temp   ○ hot   ○ cold

Comments: _____

Post-snack energy level: ○ low   ○ medium   ○ high

Medications & Supplements

Include prescription medication, over-the-counter medication & vitamin supplements.

_____   _____

_____   _____

_____   _____

_____   _____

_____   _____

Energy level | Restfulness

Today's waking energy level?
○ low   ○ medium   ○ high

# of times roused from sleep last night?
○ 1   ○ 2   ○ 3+

Last night's reflux/GERD symptoms:

_____   _____

_____   _____

Bed raised?   ○ Y   ○ N   Wedged Pillows?   ○ Y   ○ N

Last meal time? _____   Approx bedtime? _____ am pm
(Remember to give yourself at least 2-3 hours after meals before lying down.)

End-of-day notes

Noticeable change in symptoms? *(Ex: "Throat discomfort has completely disappeared.")*

_____

_____

New terms to research   Books & websites with helpful info

_____   _____

_____   _____

Additional notes:

_____

_____

_____

Breakfast

Time: _____

List the foods you ate for breakfast.

_____   _____

_____   _____

_____   _____

Drink _____   **Drink** _____
   ○ room-temp   ○ hot   ○ cold   ○ room-temp   ○ hot   ○ cold

Comments:

Physical symptoms after meal: ○ **low**   ○ **intense**   ○ **non-existent**
○ Belching   ○ Upper abdominal pain and discomfort
○ Nausea   ○ Difficulty or pain with swallowing
○ Stomach fullness or bloating   ○ Wheezing or dry cough

Other symptoms:

Post-breakfast energy level: ○ low   ○ medium   ○ high

Lunch

Time: _____

List the foods you ate for lunch.

_____   _____

_____   _____

_____   _____

Drink _____   **Drink** _____
   ○ room-temp   ○ hot   ○ cold   ○ room-temp   ○ hot   ○ cold

Comments:

Physical symptoms after meal: ○ **low**   ○ **intense**   ○ **non-existent**
○ Belching   ○ Upper abdominal pain and discomfort
○ Nausea   ○ Difficulty or pain with swallowing
○ Stomach fullness or bloating   ○ Wheezing or dry cough

Other symptoms:

Post-lunch energy level: ○ low   ○ medium   ○ high

Dinner
Time: _____

List the foods you ate for dinner.

_____   _____

_____   _____

_____   _____

Drink _____   **Drink** _____
○ room-temp ○ hot ○ cold   ○ room-temp ○ hot ○ cold

Comments: _____

Physical symptoms after meal: ○ **low** ○ **intense** ○ **non-existent**
○ Belching   ○ Upper abdominal pain and discomfort
○ Nausea   ○ Difficulty or pain with swallowing
○ Stomach fullness or bloating ○ Wheezing or dry cough

Other symptoms: _____

Post-dinner energy level: ○ low ○ medium ○ high

Snack
Time: _____

List the foods you ate as a snack.

_____   _____

Drink _____   ○ room-temp ○ hot ○ cold

Comments: _____

Post-snack energy level: ○ low ○ medium ○ high

Snack
Time: _____

List the foods you ate as a snack.

_____   _____

Drink _____   ○ room-temp ○ hot ○ cold

Comments: _____

Post-snack energy level: ○ low ○ medium ○ high

Medications & Supplements

Include prescription medication, over-the-counter medication & vitamin supplements.

_____   _____

_____   _____

_____   _____

_____   _____

_____   _____

Energy level | Restfulness

Today's waking energy level?
○ low   ○ medium   ○ high

# of times roused from sleep last night?
○ 1   ○ 2   ○ 3+

Last night's reflux/GERD symptoms:

_____   _____

_____   _____

Bed raised?   ○ Y   ○ N   Wedged Pillows?   ○ Y   ○ N

Last meal time? _____   Approx bedtime? _____   am   pm
(Remember to give yourself at least 2-3 hours after meals before lying down.)

End-of-day notes

Noticeable change in symptoms? *(Ex: "Throat discomfort has completely disappeared.")*

_____

_____

New terms to research   Books & websites with helpful info

_____   _____

_____   _____

Additional notes:

_____

_____

_____

Breakfast

Time: _____

List the foods you ate for breakfast.

_____   _____

_____   _____

_____   _____

Drink _____   **Drink** _____
 ○ room-temp ○ hot ○ cold   ○ room-temp ○ hot ○ cold

Comments: _____

Physical symptoms after meal: ○ **low**   ○ **intense**   ○ **non-existent**
 ○ Belching   ○ Upper abdominal pain and discomfort
 ○ Nausea   ○ Difficulty or pain with swallowing
 ○ Stomach fullness or bloating ○ Wheezing or dry cough

Other symptoms: _____

Post-breakfast energy level: ○ low ○ medium ○ high

Lunch

Time: _____

List the foods you ate for lunch.

_____   _____

_____   _____

_____   _____

Drink _____   **Drink** _____
 ○ room-temp ○ hot ○ cold   ○ room-temp ○ hot ○ cold

Comments: _____

Physical symptoms after meal: ○ **low**   ○ **intense**   ○ **non-existent**
 ○ Belching   ○ Upper abdominal pain and discomfort
 ○ Nausea   ○ Difficulty or pain with swallowing
 ○ Stomach fullness or bloating ○ Wheezing or dry cough

Other symptoms: _____

Post-lunch energy level: ○ low ○ medium ○ high

Dinner

Time: _____

List the foods you ate for dinner.

_____   _____

_____   _____

_____   _____

Drink _____   **Drink** _____
○ room-temp ○ hot ○ cold   ○ room-temp ○ hot ○ cold

Comments:

Physical symptoms after meal: ○ **low**   ○ **intense**   ○ **non-existent**

○ Belching   ○ Upper abdominal pain and discomfort
○ Nausea   ○ Difficulty or pain with swallowing
○ Stomach fullness or bloating   ○ Wheezing or dry cough

Other symptoms:

Post-dinner energy level: ○ low   ○ medium   ○ high

Snack

Time: _____

List the foods you ate as a snack.

_____   _____

Drink _____   ○ room-temp   ○ hot   ○ cold

Comments:

Post-snack energy level: ○ low   ○ medium   ○ high

Snack

Time: _____

List the foods you ate as a snack.

_____   _____

Drink _____   ○ room-temp   ○ hot   ○ cold

Comments:

Post-snack energy level: ○ low   ○ medium   ○ high

Medications & Supplements

Include prescription medication, over-the-counter medication & vitamin supplements.

_____   _____

_____   _____

_____   _____

_____   _____

_____   _____

Energy level | Restfulness

Today's waking energy level?
○ low   ○ medium   ○ high

# of times roused from sleep last night?
○ 1   ○ 2   ○ 3+

Last night's reflux/GERD symptoms:

_____   _____

_____   _____

Bed raised?   ○ Y   ○ N   Wedged Pillows?   ○ Y   ○ N

Last meal time? _____   Approx bedtime? _____   am   pm
(Remember to give yourself at least 2-3 hours after meals before lying down.)

End-of-day notes

Noticeable change in symptoms? _(Ex: "Throat discomfort has completely disappeared.")_

_____

_____

New terms to research   Books & websites with helpful info

_____   _____

_____   _____

Additional notes:

_____

_____

_____

Breakfast   Time: _____

List the foods you ate for breakfast.

_____   _____

_____   _____

_____   _____

Drink _____   **Drink** _____
○ room-temp ○ hot ○ cold   ○ room-temp ○ hot ○ cold

Comments:

Physical symptoms after meal: ○ **low**   ○ **intense**   ○ **non-existent**
○ Belching   ○ Upper abdominal pain and discomfort
○ Nausea   ○ Difficulty or pain with swallowing
○ Stomach fullness or bloating   ○ Wheezing or dry cough

Other symptoms:

Post-breakfast energy level: ○ low ○ medium ○ high

Lunch   Time: _____

List the foods you ate for lunch.

_____   _____

_____   _____

_____   _____

Drink _____   **Drink** _____
○ room-temp ○ hot ○ cold   ○ room-temp ○ hot ○ cold

Comments:

Physical symptoms after meal: ○ **low**   ○ **intense**   ○ **non-existent**
○ Belching   ○ Upper abdominal pain and discomfort
○ Nausea   ○ Difficulty or pain with swallowing
○ Stomach fullness or bloating   ○ Wheezing or dry cough

Other symptoms:

Post-lunch energy level: ○ low ○ medium ○ high

Dinner

Time: _____

List the foods you ate for dinner.

_____   _____

_____   _____

_____   _____

Drink _____   **Drink** _____
○ room-temp ○ hot ○ cold   ○ room-temp ○ hot ○ cold

Comments: _____

Physical symptoms after meal: ○ **low** ○ **intense** ○ **non-existent**
○ Belching   ○ Upper abdominal pain and discomfort
○ Nausea   ○ Difficulty or pain with swallowing
○ Stomach fullness or bloating   ○ Wheezing or dry cough

Other symptoms: _____

Post-dinner energy level: ○ low ○ medium ○ high

Snack

Time: _____

List the foods you ate as a snack.

_____   _____

Drink _____   ○ room-temp ○ hot ○ cold

Comments: _____

Post-snack energy level: ○ low ○ medium ○ high

Snack

Time: _____

List the foods you ate as a snack.

_____   _____

Drink _____   ○ room-temp ○ hot ○ cold

Comments: _____

Post-snack energy level: ○ low ○ medium ○ high

Medications & Supplements

Include prescription medication, over-the-counter medication & vitamin supplements.

_____   _____

_____   _____

_____   _____

_____   _____

_____   _____

Energy level | Restfulness

Today's waking energy level?
○ low   ○ medium   ○ high

# of times roused from sleep last night?
○ 1   ○ 2   ○ 3+

Last night's reflux/GERD symptoms:

_____   _____

_____   _____

Bed raised?   ○ Y   ○ N   Wedged Pillows?   ○ Y   ○ N

Last meal time? _____   Approx bedtime? _____ am pm
(Remember to give yourself at least 2-3 hours after meals before lying down.)

End-of-day notes

Noticeable change in symptoms? *(Ex: "Throat discomfort has completely disappeared.")*

_____

_____

New terms to research   Books & websites with helpful info

_____   _____

_____   _____

Additional notes:

_____

_____

_____

Breakfast   Time: _____

List the foods you ate for breakfast.

_____   _____

_____   _____

_____   _____

Drink _____   **Drink** _____
  ○ room-temp ○ hot ○ cold   ○ room-temp ○ hot ○ cold

Comments: _____

Physical symptoms after meal: ○ **low** ○ **intense** ○ **non-existent**
○ Belching   ○ Upper abdominal pain and discomfort
○ Nausea   ○ Difficulty or pain with swallowing
○ Stomach fullness or bloating   ○ Wheezing or dry cough

Other symptoms: _____

Post-breakfast energy level: ○ low ○ medium ○ high

Lunch   Time: _____

List the foods you ate for lunch.

_____   _____

_____   _____

_____   _____

Drink _____   **Drink** _____
  ○ room-temp ○ hot ○ cold   ○ room-temp ○ hot ○ cold

Comments: _____

Physical symptoms after meal: ○ **low** ○ **intense** ○ **non-existent**
○ Belching   ○ Upper abdominal pain and discomfort
○ Nausea   ○ Difficulty or pain with swallowing
○ Stomach fullness or bloating   ○ Wheezing or dry cough

Other symptoms: _____

Post-lunch energy level: ○ low ○ medium ○ high

Dinner

Time: _____

List the foods you ate for dinner.

_____   _____

_____   _____

_____   _____

Drink _____   **Drink** _____
○ room-temp   ○ hot   ○ cold   ○ room-temp   ○ hot   ○ cold

Comments: _____

Physical symptoms after meal: ○ **low**   ○ **intense**   ○ **non-existent**
○ Belching   ○ Upper abdominal pain and discomfort
○ Nausea   ○ Difficulty or pain with swallowing
○ Stomach fullness or bloating   ○ Wheezing or dry cough

Other symptoms: _____

Post-dinner energy level: ○ low   ○ medium   ○ high

Snack

Time: _____

List the foods you ate as a snack.

_____   _____

Drink _____   ○ room-temp   ○ hot   ○ cold

Comments: _____

Post-snack energy level: ○ low   ○ medium   ○ high

Snack

Time: _____

List the foods you ate as a snack.

_____   _____

Drink _____   ○ room-temp   ○ hot   ○ cold

Comments: _____

Post-snack energy level: ○ low   ○ medium   ○ high

Medications & Supplements

Include prescription medication, over-the-counter medication & vitamin supplements.

_____   _____

_____   _____

_____   _____

_____   _____

_____   _____

Energy level | Restfulness

Today's waking energy level?
○ low   ○ medium   ○ high

# of times roused from sleep last night?
○ 1   ○ 2   ○ 3+

Last night's reflux/GERD symptoms:

_____   _____

_____   _____

Bed raised?   ○ Y   ○ N   Wedged Pillows?   ○ Y   ○ N

Last meal time? _____   Approx bedtime? _____   am pm
(Remember to give yourself at least 2-3 hours after meals before lying down.)

End-of-day notes

Noticeable change in symptoms? *(Ex: "Throat discomfort has completely disappeared.")*

_____

_____

New terms to research   Books & websites with helpful info

_____   _____

_____   _____

Additional notes:

_____

_____

_____

DATE	

Breakfast
Time: _____

List the foods you ate for breakfast.

_____   _____

_____   _____

_____   _____

Drink _____   **Drink** _____
○ room-temp ○ hot ○ cold   ○ room-temp ○ hot ○ cold

Comments:

Physical symptoms after meal: ○ **low** ○ **intense** ○ **non-existent**
○ Belching   ○ Upper abdominal pain and discomfort
○ Nausea   ○ Difficulty or pain with swallowing
○ Stomach fullness or bloating   ○ Wheezing or dry cough

Other symptoms:

Post-breakfast energy level: ○ low ○ medium ○ high

Lunch
Time: _____

List the foods you ate for lunch.

_____   _____

_____   _____

_____   _____

Drink _____   **Drink** _____
○ room-temp ○ hot ○ cold   ○ room-temp ○ hot ○ cold

Comments:

Physical symptoms after meal: ○ **low** ○ **intense** ○ **non-existent**
○ Belching   ○ Upper abdominal pain and discomfort
○ Nausea   ○ Difficulty or pain with swallowing
○ Stomach fullness or bloating   ○ Wheezing or dry cough

Other symptoms:

Post-lunch energy level: ○ low ○ medium ○ high

Dinner

Time: _____

List the foods you ate for dinner.

_____   _____

_____   _____

_____   _____

Drink _____   **Drink** _____
  ○ room-temp   ○ hot   ○ cold   ○ room-temp   ○ hot   ○ cold

Comments: _____

Physical symptoms after meal: ○ **low**   ○ **intense**   ○ **non-existent**
○ Belching   ○ Upper abdominal pain and discomfort
○ Nausea   ○ Difficulty or pain with swallowing
○ Stomach fullness or bloating   ○ Wheezing or dry cough

Other symptoms: _____

Post-dinner energy level: ○ low   ○ medium   ○ high

Snack

Time: _____

List the foods you ate as a snack.

_____   _____

Drink _____   ○ room-temp   ○ hot   ○ cold

Comments: _____

Post-snack energy level: ○ low   ○ medium   ○ high

Snack

Time: _____

List the foods you ate as a snack.

_____   _____

Drink _____   ○ room-temp   ○ hot   ○ cold

Comments: _____

Post-snack energy level: ○ low   ○ medium   ○ high

Medications & Supplements

Include prescription medication, over-the-counter medication & vitamin supplements.

_____   _____

_____   _____

_____   _____

_____   _____

_____   _____

Energy level | Restfulness

Today's waking energy level?
○ low   ○ medium   ○ high

# of times roused from sleep last night?
○ 1   ○ 2   ○ 3+

Last night's reflux/GERD symptoms:

_____   _____

_____   _____

Bed raised?   ○ Y   ○ N   Wedged Pillows?   ○ Y   ○ N

Last meal time? _____   Approx bedtime? _____ am pm
(Remember to give yourself at least 2-3 hours after meals before lying down.)

End-of-day notes

Noticeable change in symptoms? *(Ex: "Throat discomfort has completely disappeared.")*

_____

_____

New terms to research   Books & websites with helpful info

_____   _____

_____   _____

Additional notes:

_____

_____

_____

Breakfast

Time: _____

List the foods you ate for breakfast.

_____   _____

_____   _____

_____   _____

Drink _____   **Drink** _____
  ○ room-temp   ○ hot   ○ cold   ○ room-temp   ○ hot   ○ cold

Comments: _____

Physical symptoms after meal: ○ **low**   ○ **intense**   ○ **non-existent**
○ Belching   ○ Upper abdominal pain and discomfort
○ Nausea   ○ Difficulty or pain with swallowing
○ Stomach fullness or bloating   ○ Wheezing or dry cough

Other symptoms: _____

Post-breakfast energy level: ○ low   ○ medium   ○ high

Lunch

Time: _____

List the foods you ate for lunch.

_____   _____

_____   _____

_____   _____

Drink _____   **Drink** _____
  ○ room-temp   ○ hot   ○ cold   ○ room-temp   ○ hot   ○ cold

Comments: _____

Physical symptoms after meal: ○ **low**   ○ **intense**   ○ **non-existent**
○ Belching   ○ Upper abdominal pain and discomfort
○ Nausea   ○ Difficulty or pain with swallowing
○ Stomach fullness or bloating   ○ Wheezing or dry cough

Other symptoms: _____

Post-lunch energy level: ○ low   ○ medium   ○ high

Dinner

Time: _____

List the foods you ate for dinner.

_____   _____

_____   _____

_____   _____

Drink _____   **Drink** _____
○ room-temp   ○ hot   ○ cold   ○ room-temp   ○ hot   ○ cold

Comments: _____

Physical symptoms after meal: ○ **low**   ○ **intense**   ○ **non-existent**
○ Belching   ○ Upper abdominal pain and discomfort
○ Nausea   ○ Difficulty or pain with swallowing
○ Stomach fullness or bloating   ○ Wheezing or dry cough

Other symptoms: _____

Post-dinner energy level: ○ low   ○ medium   ○ high

Snack

Time: _____

List the foods you ate as a snack.

_____   _____

Drink _____   ○ room-temp   ○ hot   ○ cold

Comments: _____

Post-snack energy level: ○ low   ○ medium   ○ high

Snack

Time: _____

List the foods you ate as a snack.

_____   _____

Drink _____   ○ room-temp   ○ hot   ○ cold

Comments: _____

Post-snack energy level: ○ low   ○ medium   ○ high

Medications & Supplements

Include prescription medication, over-the-counter medication & vitamin supplements.

_____   _____

_____   _____

_____   _____

_____   _____

_____

Energy level | Restfulness

Today's waking energy level?
○ low   ○ medium   ○ high

# of times roused from sleep last night?
○ 1   ○ 2   ○ 3+

Last night's reflux/GERD symptoms:

_____   _____

_____   _____

Bed raised?   ○ Y   ○ N   Wedged Pillows?   ○ Y   ○ N

Last meal time? _____   Approx bedtime? _____ am pm
(Remember to give yourself at least 2-3 hours after meals before lying down.)

End-of-day notes

Noticeable change in symptoms? _(Ex: "Throat discomfort has completely disappeared.")_

_____

_____

New terms to research   Books & websites with helpful info

_____   _____

_____   _____

Additional notes:

_____

_____

_____

Breakfast
Time: _____

List the foods you ate for breakfast.

_____   _____

_____   _____

_____   _____

Drink _____   **Drink** _____
  ○ room-temp ○ hot ○ cold   ○ room-temp ○ hot ○ cold

Comments:

Physical symptoms after meal: ○ **low** ○ **intense** ○ **non-existent**
○ Belching   ○ Upper abdominal pain and discomfort
○ Nausea   ○ Difficulty or pain with swallowing
○ Stomach fullness or bloating   ○ Wheezing or dry cough

Other symptoms:

Post-breakfast energy level: ○ low ○ medium ○ high

Lunch
Time: _____

List the foods you ate for lunch.

_____   _____

_____   _____

_____   _____

Drink _____   **Drink** _____
  ○ room-temp ○ hot ○ cold   ○ room-temp ○ hot ○ cold

Comments:

Physical symptoms after meal: ○ **low** ○ **intense** ○ **non-existent**
○ Belching   ○ Upper abdominal pain and discomfort
○ Nausea   ○ Difficulty or pain with swallowing
○ Stomach fullness or bloating   ○ Wheezing or dry cough

Other symptoms:

Post-lunch energy level: ○ low ○ medium ○ high

Dinner

Time: _____

List the foods you ate for dinner.

_____   _____

_____   _____

_____   _____

Drink _____   **Drink** _____

    ○ room-temp   ○ hot   ○ cold   ○ room-temp   ○ hot   ○ cold

Comments: _____

Physical symptoms after meal: ○ **low**   ○ **intense**   ○ **non-existent**
○ Belching   ○ Upper abdominal pain and discomfort
○ Nausea   ○ Difficulty or pain with swallowing
○ Stomach fullness or bloating   ○ Wheezing or dry cough

Other symptoms: _____

Post-dinner energy level: ○ low   ○ medium   ○ high

Snack

Time: _____

List the foods you ate as a snack.

_____   _____

Drink _____   ○ room-temp   ○ hot   ○ cold

Comments: _____

Post-snack energy level: ○ low   ○ medium   ○ high

Snack

Time: _____

List the foods you ate as a snack.

_____   _____

Drink _____   ○ room-temp   ○ hot   ○ cold

Comments: _____

Post-snack energy level: ○ low   ○ medium   ○ high

Medications & Supplements

Include prescription medication, over-the-counter medication & vitamin supplements.

_____   _____

_____   _____

_____   _____

_____   _____

_____   _____

Energy level | Restfulness

Today's waking energy level?
○ low   ○ medium   ○ high

# of times roused from sleep last night?
○ 1   ○ 2   ○ 3+

Last night's reflux/GERD symptoms:

_____   _____

_____   _____

Bed raised?   ○ Y   ○ N   Wedged Pillows?   ○ Y   ○ N

Last meal time? _____   Approx bedtime? _____   am   pm
(Remember to give yourself at least 2-3 hours after meals before lying down.)

End-of-day notes

Noticeable change in symptoms? _(Ex: "Throat discomfort has completely disappeared.")_

_____

_____

New terms to research   Books & websites with helpful info

_____   _____

_____   _____

Additional notes:

_____

_____

_____

DATE

Breakfast
Time: _____

List the foods you ate for breakfast.

_____   _____

_____   _____

_____   _____

Drink _____   **Drink** _____
○ room-temp ○ hot ○ cold   ○ room-temp ○ hot ○ cold

Comments: _____

Physical symptoms after meal: ○ **low** ○ **intense** ○ **non-existent**
○ Belching   ○ Upper abdominal pain and discomfort
○ Nausea   ○ Difficulty or pain with swallowing
○ Stomach fullness or bloating ○ Wheezing or dry cough

Other symptoms: _____

Post-breakfast energy level: ○ low ○ medium ○ high

Lunch
Time: _____

List the foods you ate for lunch.

_____   _____

_____   _____

_____   _____

Drink _____   **Drink** _____
○ room-temp ○ hot ○ cold   ○ room-temp ○ hot ○ cold

Comments: _____

Physical symptoms after meal: ○ **low** ○ **intense** ○ **non-existent**
○ Belching   ○ Upper abdominal pain and discomfort
○ Nausea   ○ Difficulty or pain with swallowing
○ Stomach fullness or bloating ○ Wheezing or dry cough

Other symptoms: _____

Post-lunch energy level: ○ low ○ medium ○ high

Dinner

Time: _____

List the foods you ate for dinner.

_____   _____

_____   _____

_____   _____

Drink _____   **Drink** _____
○ room-temp ○ hot ○ cold   ○ room-temp ○ hot ○ cold

Comments: _____

Physical symptoms after meal: ○ **low**   ○ **intense**   ○ **non-existent**
○ Belching   ○ Upper abdominal pain and discomfort
○ Nausea   ○ Difficulty or pain with swallowing
○ Stomach fullness or bloating   ○ Wheezing or dry cough

Other symptoms: _____

Post-dinner energy level: ○ low   ○ medium   ○ high

Snack

Time: _____

List the foods you ate as a snack.

_____   _____

Drink _____   ○ room-temp   ○ hot   ○ cold

Comments: _____

Post-snack energy level: ○ low   ○ medium   ○ high

Snack

Time: _____

List the foods you ate as a snack.

_____   _____

Drink _____   ○ room-temp   ○ hot   ○ cold

Comments: _____

Post-snack energy level: ○ low   ○ medium   ○ high

Medications & Supplements

Include prescription medication, over-the-counter medication & vitamin supplements.

_____   _____

_____   _____

_____   _____

_____   _____

_____   _____

Energy level | Restfulness

Today's waking energy level?
○ low   ○ medium   ○ high

# of times roused from sleep last night?
○ 1   ○ 2   ○ 3+

Last night's reflux/GERD symptoms:

_____   _____

_____   _____

Bed raised?   ○ Y   ○ N   Wedged Pillows?   ○ Y   ○ N

Last meal time? _____   Approx bedtime? _____ am pm
(Remember to give yourself at least 2-3 hours after meals before lying down.)

End-of-day notes

Noticeable change in symptoms? *(Ex: "Throat discomfort has completely disappeared.")*

_____

_____

New terms to research   Books & websites with helpful info

_____   _____

_____   _____

Additional notes:

_____

_____

_____

DATE	

Breakfast   Time: _____

List the foods you ate for breakfast.

_____   _____

_____   _____

_____   _____

Drink _____   **Drink** _____
○ room-temp   ○ hot   ○ cold   ○ room-temp   ○ hot   ○ cold

Comments:

Physical symptoms after meal: ○ **low**   ○ **intense**   ○ **non-existent**
○ Belching   ○ Upper abdominal pain and discomfort
○ Nausea   ○ Difficulty or pain with swallowing
○ Stomach fullness or bloating ○ Wheezing or dry cough

Other symptoms:

Post-breakfast energy level: ○ low   ○ medium   ○ high

Lunch   Time: _____

List the foods you ate for lunch.

_____   _____

_____   _____

_____   _____

Drink _____   **Drink** _____
○ room-temp   ○ hot   ○ cold   ○ room-temp   ○ hot   ○ cold

Comments:

Physical symptoms after meal: ○ **low**   ○ **intense**   ○ **non-existent**
○ Belching   ○ Upper abdominal pain and discomfort
○ Nausea   ○ Difficulty or pain with swallowing
○ Stomach fullness or bloating ○ Wheezing or dry cough

Other symptoms:

Post-lunch energy level: ○ low   ○ medium   ○ high

Dinner

Time: _____

List the foods you ate for dinner.

_____   _____

_____   _____

_____   _____

Drink _____   **Drink** _____
    ○ room-temp   ○ hot   ○ cold   ○ room-temp   ○ hot   ○ cold

Comments: _____

Physical symptoms after meal: ○ **low**   ○ **intense**   ○ **non-existent**
○ Belching   ○ Upper abdominal pain and discomfort
○ Nausea   ○ Difficulty or pain with swallowing
○ Stomach fullness or bloating   ○ Wheezing or dry cough

Other symptoms: _____

Post-dinner energy level: ○ low   ○ medium   ○ high

Snack

Time: _____

List the foods you ate as a snack.

_____   _____

Drink _____   ○ room-temp   ○ hot   ○ cold

Comments: _____

Post-snack energy level: ○ low   ○ medium   ○ high

Snack

Time: _____

List the foods you ate as a snack.

_____   _____

Drink _____   ○ room-temp   ○ hot   ○ cold

Comments: _____

Post-snack energy level: ○ low   ○ medium   ○ high

Medications & Supplements

Include prescription medication, over-the-counter medication & vitamin supplements.

_____   _____

_____   _____

_____   _____

_____   _____

_____   _____

Energy level | Restfulness

Today's waking energy level?
○ low   ○ medium   ○ high

# of times roused from sleep last night?
○ 1   ○ 2   ○ 3+

Last night's reflux/GERD symptoms:

_____   _____

_____   _____

Bed raised?   ○ Y   ○ N   Wedged Pillows?   ○ Y   ○ N

Last meal time? _____   Approx bedtime? _____   am   pm

(Remember to give yourself at least 2-3 hours after meals before lying down.)

End-of-day notes

Noticeable change in symptoms? *(Ex: "Throat discomfort has completely disappeared.")*

_____

_____

New terms to research   Books & websites with helpful info

_____   _____

_____   _____

Additional notes:

_____

_____

_____

Breakfast   Time: _____

List the foods you ate for breakfast.

_____   _____

_____   _____

_____   _____

Drink _____   **Drink** _____
○ room-temp ○ hot ○ cold   ○ room-temp ○ hot ○ cold

Comments: _____

Physical symptoms after meal: ○ **low**   ○ **intense**   ○ **non-existent**
○ Belching   ○ Upper abdominal pain and discomfort
○ Nausea   ○ Difficulty or pain with swallowing
○ Stomach fullness or bloating ○ Wheezing or dry cough

Other symptoms: _____

Post-breakfast energy level: ○ low   ○ medium   ○ high

Lunch   Time: _____

List the foods you ate for lunch.

_____   _____

_____   _____

_____   _____

Drink _____   **Drink** _____
○ room-temp ○ hot ○ cold   ○ room-temp ○ hot ○ cold

Comments: _____

Physical symptoms after meal: ○ **low**   ○ **intense**   ○ **non-existent**
○ Belching   ○ Upper abdominal pain and discomfort
○ Nausea   ○ Difficulty or pain with swallowing
○ Stomach fullness or bloating ○ Wheezing or dry cough

Other symptoms: _____

Post-lunch energy level: ○ low   ○ medium   ○ high

Dinner

Time: _____

List the foods you ate for dinner.

_____   _____

_____   _____

_____   _____

Drink _____   **Drink** _____
○ room-temp ○ hot ○ cold   ○ room-temp ○ hot ○ cold

Comments: _____

Physical symptoms after meal: ○ **low** ○ **intense** ○ **non-existent**
○ Belching   ○ Upper abdominal pain and discomfort
○ Nausea   ○ Difficulty or pain with swallowing
○ Stomach fullness or bloating ○ Wheezing or dry cough

Other symptoms: _____

Post-dinner energy level: ○ low ○ medium ○ high

Snack

Time: _____

List the foods you ate as a snack.

_____   _____

Drink _____   ○ room-temp ○ hot ○ cold

Comments: _____

Post-snack energy level: ○ low ○ medium ○ high

Snack

Time: _____

List the foods you ate as a snack.

_____   _____

Drink _____   ○ room-temp ○ hot ○ cold

Comments: _____

Post-snack energy level: ○ low ○ medium ○ high

Medications & Supplements

Include prescription medication, over-the-counter medication & vitamin supplements.

_____   _____

_____   _____

_____   _____

_____   _____

_____   _____

Energy level | Restfulness

Today's waking energy level?
○ low   ○ medium   ○ high

# of times roused from sleep last night?
○ 1   ○ 2   ○ 3+

Last night's reflux/GERD symptoms:

_____   _____

_____   _____

Bed raised?   ○ Y   ○ N   Wedged Pillows?   ○ Y   ○ N

Last meal time? _____   Approx bedtime? _____ am pm

(Remember to give yourself at least 2-3 hours after meals before lying down.)

End-of-day notes

Noticeable change in symptoms? *(Ex: "Throat discomfort has completely disappeared.")*

_____

_____

New terms to research   Books & websites with helpful info

_____   _____

_____   _____

Additional notes:

_____

_____

_____

Breakfast

Time: _____

List the foods you ate for breakfast.

_____   _____

_____   _____

_____   _____

Drink _____   **Drink** _____
○ room-temp   ○ hot   ○ cold   ○ room-temp   ○ hot   ○ cold

Comments:

_____

Physical symptoms after meal: ○ **low**   ○ **intense**   ○ **non-existent**
○ Belching   ○ Upper abdominal pain and discomfort
○ Nausea   ○ Difficulty or pain with swallowing
○ Stomach fullness or bloating   ○ Wheezing or dry cough

Other symptoms:

Post-breakfast energy level: ○ low   ○ medium   ○ high

Lunch

Time: _____

List the foods you ate for lunch.

_____   _____

_____   _____

_____   _____

Drink _____   **Drink** _____
○ room-temp   ○ hot   ○ cold   ○ room-temp   ○ hot   ○ cold

Comments:

_____

Physical symptoms after meal: ○ **low**   ○ **intense**   ○ **non-existent**
○ Belching   ○ Upper abdominal pain and discomfort
○ Nausea   ○ Difficulty or pain with swallowing
○ Stomach fullness or bloating   ○ Wheezing or dry cough

Other symptoms:

Post-lunch energy level: ○ low   ○ medium   ○ high

Dinner

Time: _____

List the foods you ate for dinner.

_____   _____

_____   _____

_____   _____

Drink _____   **Drink** _____
  ○ room-temp   ○ hot   ○ cold   ○ room-temp   ○ hot   ○ cold

Comments: _____

Physical symptoms after meal: ○ **low**   ○ **intense**   ○ **non-existent**
○ Belching   ○ Upper abdominal pain and discomfort
○ Nausea   ○ Difficulty or pain with swallowing
○ Stomach fullness or bloating   ○ Wheezing or dry cough

Other symptoms: _____

Post-dinner energy level: ○ low   ○ medium   ○ high

Snack

Time: _____

List the foods you ate as a snack.

_____   _____

Drink _____   ○ room-temp   ○ hot   ○ cold

Comments: _____

Post-snack energy level: ○ low   ○ medium   ○ high

Snack

Time: _____

List the foods you ate as a snack.

_____   _____

Drink _____   ○ room-temp   ○ hot   ○ cold

Comments: _____

Post-snack energy level: ○ low   ○ medium   ○ high

Medications & Supplements

Include prescription medication, over-the-counter medication & vitamin supplements.

_____   _____

_____   _____

_____   _____

_____   _____

_____   _____

Energy level | Restfulness

Today's waking energy level?
○ low   ○ medium   ○ high

# of times roused from sleep last night?
○ 1   ○ 2   ○ 3+

Last night's reflux/GERD symptoms:

_____   _____

_____   _____

Bed raised?   ○ Y   ○ N   Wedged Pillows?   ○ Y   ○ N

Last meal time? _____   Approx bedtime? _____ am pm
(Remember to give yourself at least 2-3 hours after meals before lying down.)

End-of-day notes

Noticeable change in symptoms? _(Ex: "Throat discomfort has completely disappeared.")_

_____

_____

New terms to research   Books & websites with helpful info

_____   _____

_____   _____

Additional notes:

_____

_____

_____

Breakfast   Time: _____

List the foods you ate for breakfast.

_____   _____

_____   _____

_____   _____

Drink _____   **Drink** _____
○ room-temp ○ hot ○ cold   ○ room-temp ○ hot ○ cold

Comments: _____

Physical symptoms after meal: ○ **low**   ○ **intense**   ○ **non-existent**
○ Belching   ○ Upper abdominal pain and discomfort
○ Nausea   ○ Difficulty or pain with swallowing
○ Stomach fullness or bloating ○ Wheezing or dry cough

Other symptoms: _____

Post-breakfast energy level: ○ low   ○ medium   ○ high

Lunch   Time: _____

List the foods you ate for lunch.

_____   _____

_____   _____

_____   _____

Drink _____   **Drink** _____
○ room-temp ○ hot ○ cold   ○ room-temp ○ hot ○ cold

Comments: _____

Physical symptoms after meal: ○ **low**   ○ **intense**   ○ **non-existent**
○ Belching   ○ Upper abdominal pain and discomfort
○ Nausea   ○ Difficulty or pain with swallowing
○ Stomach fullness or bloating ○ Wheezing or dry cough

Other symptoms: _____

Post-lunch energy level: ○ low   ○ medium   ○ high

Dinner

Time: _____

List the foods you ate for dinner.

_____   _____

_____   _____

_____   _____

Drink _____   **Drink** _____
○ room-temp ○ hot ○ cold   ○ room-temp ○ hot ○ cold

Comments: _____

Physical symptoms after meal: ○ **low**   ○ **intense**   ○ **non-existent**
○ Belching   ○ Upper abdominal pain and discomfort
○ Nausea   ○ Difficulty or pain with swallowing
○ Stomach fullness or bloating   ○ Wheezing or dry cough

Other symptoms: _____

Post-dinner energy level: ○ low   ○ medium   ○ high

Snack

Time: _____

List the foods you ate as a snack.

_____   _____

Drink _____   ○ room-temp   ○ hot   ○ cold

Comments: _____

Post-snack energy level: ○ low   ○ medium   ○ high

Snack

Time: _____

List the foods you ate as a snack.

_____   _____

Drink _____   ○ room-temp   ○ hot   ○ cold

Comments: _____

Post-snack energy level: ○ low   ○ medium   ○ high

Medications & Supplements

Include prescription medication, over-the-counter medication & vitamin supplements.

_____   _____

_____   _____

_____   _____

_____   _____

_____   _____

Energy level | Restfulness

Today's waking energy level?
○ low   ○ medium   ○ high

# of times roused from sleep last night?
○ 1   ○ 2   ○ 3+

Last night's reflux/GERD symptoms:

_____   _____

_____   _____

Bed raised?   ○ Y   ○ N   Wedged Pillows?   ○ Y   ○ N

Last meal time? _____   Approx bedtime? _____   am   pm
(Remember to give yourself at least 2-3 hours after meals before lying down.)

End-of-day notes

Noticeable change in symptoms? *(Ex: "Throat discomfort has completely disappeared.")*

_____

_____

New terms to research   Books & websites with helpful info

_____   _____

_____   _____

Additional notes:

_____

_____

_____

Breakfast   Time: _____

List the foods you ate for breakfast.

_____   _____

_____   _____

_____   _____

Drink _____   **Drink** _____
○ room-temp ○ hot ○ cold   ○ room-temp ○ hot ○ cold

Comments:

Physical symptoms after meal: ○ **low** ○ **intense** ○ **non-existent**
○ Belching   ○ Upper abdominal pain and discomfort
○ Nausea   ○ Difficulty or pain with swallowing
○ Stomach fullness or bloating   ○ Wheezing or dry cough

Other symptoms:

Post-breakfast energy level: ○ low ○ medium ○ high

Lunch   Time: _____

List the foods you ate for lunch.

_____   _____

_____   _____

_____   _____

Drink _____   **Drink** _____
○ room-temp ○ hot ○ cold   ○ room-temp ○ hot ○ cold

Comments:

Physical symptoms after meal: ○ **low** ○ **intense** ○ **non-existent**
○ Belching   ○ Upper abdominal pain and discomfort
○ Nausea   ○ Difficulty or pain with swallowing
○ Stomach fullness or bloating   ○ Wheezing or dry cough

Other symptoms:

Post-lunch energy level: ○ low ○ medium ○ high

Dinner

Time: _____

List the foods you ate for dinner.

_____   _____

_____   _____

Drink _____   **Drink** _____
  ○ room-temp ○ hot ○ cold   ○ room-temp ○ hot ○ cold

Comments: _____

Physical symptoms after meal: ○ **low** ○ **intense** ○ **non-existent**
○ Belching   ○ Upper abdominal pain and discomfort
○ Nausea   ○ Difficulty or pain with swallowing
○ Stomach fullness or bloating ○ Wheezing or dry cough

Other symptoms: _____

Post-dinner energy level: ○ low ○ medium ○ high

Snack

Time: _____

List the foods you ate as a snack.

_____   _____

Drink _____   ○ room-temp ○ hot ○ cold

Comments: _____

Post-snack energy level: ○ low ○ medium ○ high

Snack

Time: _____

List the foods you ate as a snack.

_____   _____

Drink _____   ○ room-temp ○ hot ○ cold

Comments: _____

Post-snack energy level: ○ low ○ medium ○ high

Medications & Supplements

Include prescription medication, over-the-counter medication & vitamin supplements.

_____   _____

_____   _____

_____   _____

_____   _____

_____   _____

Energy level | Restfulness

Today's waking energy level?
○ low   ○ medium   ○ high

# of times roused from sleep last night?
○ 1   ○ 2   ○ 3+

Last night's reflux/GERD symptoms:

_____   _____

_____   _____

Bed raised?   ○ Y   ○ N   Wedged Pillows?   ○ Y   ○ N

Last meal time? _____   Approx bedtime? _____   am   pm
(Remember to give yourself at least 2-3 hours after meals before lying down.)

End-of-day notes

Noticeable change in symptoms? _(Ex: "Throat discomfort has completely disappeared.")_

_____

_____

New terms to research   Books & websites with helpful info

_____   _____

_____   _____

Additional notes:

_____

_____

_____

Breakfast   Time: _____

List the foods you ate for breakfast.

_____   _____

_____   _____

_____   _____

Drink _____   **Drink** _____
   ○ room-temp ○ hot ○ cold   ○ room-temp ○ hot ○ cold

Comments: _____

Physical symptoms after meal: ○ **low**   ○ **intense**   ○ **non-existent**
○ Belching   ○ Upper abdominal pain and discomfort
○ Nausea   ○ Difficulty or pain with swallowing
○ Stomach fullness or bloating   ○ Wheezing or dry cough

Other symptoms: _____

Post-breakfast energy level: ○ low   ○ medium   ○ high

Lunch   Time: _____

List the foods you ate for lunch.

_____   _____

_____   _____

_____   _____

Drink _____   **Drink** _____
   ○ room-temp ○ hot ○ cold   ○ room-temp ○ hot ○ cold

Comments: _____

Physical symptoms after meal: ○ **low**   ○ **intense**   ○ **non-existent**
○ Belching   ○ Upper abdominal pain and discomfort
○ Nausea   ○ Difficulty or pain with swallowing
○ Stomach fullness or bloating   ○ Wheezing or dry cough

Other symptoms: _____

Post-lunch energy level: ○ low   ○ medium   ○ high

Dinner

Time: _____

List the foods you ate for dinner.

_____   _____

_____   _____

_____   _____

Drink _____   **Drink** _____
○ room-temp ○ hot ○ cold   ○ room-temp ○ hot ○ cold

Comments:

Physical symptoms after meal: ○ **low** ○ **intense** ○ **non-existent**
○ Belching   ○ Upper abdominal pain and discomfort
○ Nausea   ○ Difficulty or pain with swallowing
○ Stomach fullness or bloating   ○ Wheezing or dry cough

Other symptoms:

Post-dinner energy level: ○ low ○ medium ○ high

Snack

Time: _____

List the foods you ate as a snack.

_____   _____

Drink _____ ○ room-temp ○ hot ○ cold

Comments:

Post-snack energy level: ○ low ○ medium ○ high

Snack

Time: _____

List the foods you ate as a snack.

_____   _____

Drink _____ ○ room-temp ○ hot ○ cold

Comments:

Post-snack energy level: ○ low ○ medium ○ high

Medications & Supplements

Include prescription medication, over-the-counter medication & vitamin supplements.

_____   _____

_____   _____

_____   _____

_____   _____

_____   _____

Energy level | Restfulness

Today's waking energy level?
○ low   ○ medium   ○ high

# of times roused from sleep last night?
○ 1   ○ 2   ○ 3+

Last night's reflux/GERD symptoms:

_____   _____

_____   _____

Bed raised?   ○ Y   ○ N   Wedged Pillows?   ○ Y   ○ N

Last meal time? _____   Approx bedtime? _____ am pm
(Remember to give yourself at least 2-3 hours after meals before lying down.)

End-of-day notes

Noticeable change in symptoms? _(Ex: "Throat discomfort has completely disappeared.")_

_____

_____

New terms to research   Books & websites with helpful info

_____   _____

_____   _____

Additional notes:

_____

_____

_____

Breakfast
Time: _____

List the foods you ate for breakfast.

_____   _____

_____   _____

_____   _____

Drink _____   **Drink** _____
○ room-temp ○ hot ○ cold   ○ room-temp ○ hot ○ cold

Comments:

Physical symptoms after meal: ○ **low** ○ **intense** ○ **non-existent**
○ Belching   ○ Upper abdominal pain and discomfort
○ Nausea   ○ Difficulty or pain with swallowing
○ Stomach fullness or bloating   ○ Wheezing or dry cough

Other symptoms:

Post-breakfast energy level: ○ low ○ medium ○ high

Lunch
Time: _____

List the foods you ate for lunch.

_____   _____

_____   _____

_____   _____

Drink _____   **Drink** _____
○ room-temp ○ hot ○ cold   ○ room-temp ○ hot ○ cold

Comments:

Physical symptoms after meal: ○ **low** ○ **intense** ○ **non-existent**
○ Belching   ○ Upper abdominal pain and discomfort
○ Nausea   ○ Difficulty or pain with swallowing
○ Stomach fullness or bloating   ○ Wheezing or dry cough

Other symptoms:

Post-lunch energy level: ○ low ○ medium ○ high

Dinner

Time: _____

List the foods you ate for dinner.

_____   _____

_____   _____

_____   _____

Drink _____   **Drink** _____
  ○ room-temp   ○ hot   ○ cold   ○ room-temp   ○ hot   ○ cold

Comments: _____

Physical symptoms after meal: ○ **low**   ○ **intense**   ○ **non-existent**
○ Belching   ○ Upper abdominal pain and discomfort
○ Nausea   ○ Difficulty or pain with swallowing
○ Stomach fullness or bloating ○ Wheezing or dry cough

Other symptoms: _____

Post-dinner energy level: ○ low   ○ medium   ○ high

Snack

Time: _____

List the foods you ate as a snack.

_____   _____

Drink _____   ○ room-temp   ○ hot   ○ cold

Comments: _____

Post-snack energy level: ○ low   ○ medium   ○ high

Snack

Time: _____

List the foods you ate as a snack.

_____   _____

Drink _____   ○ room-temp   ○ hot   ○ cold

Comments: _____

Post-snack energy level: ○ low   ○ medium   ○ high

Medications & Supplements

Include prescription medication, over-the-counter medication & vitamin supplements.

_____   _____

_____   _____

_____   _____

_____   _____

_____   _____

Energy level | Restfulness

Today's waking energy level?
○ low   ○ medium   ○ high

# of times roused from sleep last night?
○ 1   ○ 2   ○ 3+

Last night's reflux/GERD symptoms:

_____   _____

_____   _____

Bed raised?   ○ Y   ○ N   Wedged Pillows?   ○ Y   ○ N

Last meal time? _____   Approx bedtime? _____   am   pm
(Remember to give yourself at least 2-3 hours after meals before lying down.)

End-of-day notes

Noticeable change in symptoms? _(Ex: "Throat discomfort has completely disappeared.")_

_____

_____

New terms to research   Books & websites with helpful info

_____   _____

_____   _____

Additional notes:

_____

_____

_____

Breakfast
Time: _____

List the foods you ate for breakfast.

_____   _____

_____   _____

_____   _____

Drink _____   **Drink** _____
○ room-temp   ○ hot   ○ cold   ○ room-temp   ○ hot   ○ cold

Comments: _____

Physical symptoms after meal: ○ **low**   ○ **intense**   ○ **non-existent**
○ Belching   ○ Upper abdominal pain and discomfort
○ Nausea   ○ Difficulty or pain with swallowing
○ Stomach fullness or bloating   ○ Wheezing or dry cough

Other symptoms: _____

Post-breakfast energy level: ○ low   ○ medium   ○ high

Lunch
Time: _____

List the foods you ate for lunch.

_____   _____

_____   _____

_____   _____

Drink _____   **Drink** _____
○ room-temp   ○ hot   ○ cold   ○ room-temp   ○ hot   ○ cold

Comments: _____

Physical symptoms after meal: ○ **low**   ○ **intense**   ○ **non-existent**
○ Belching   ○ Upper abdominal pain and discomfort
○ Nausea   ○ Difficulty or pain with swallowing
○ Stomach fullness or bloating   ○ Wheezing or dry cough

Other symptoms: _____

Post-lunch energy level: ○ low   ○ medium   ○ high

Dinner

Time: _____

List the foods you ate for dinner.

_____   _____

_____   _____

_____   _____

Drink _____   **Drink** _____
○ room-temp ○ hot ○ cold   ○ room-temp ○ hot ○ cold

Comments: _____

Physical symptoms after meal: ○ **low** ○ **intense** ○ **non-existent**
○ Belching   ○ Upper abdominal pain and discomfort
○ Nausea   ○ Difficulty or pain with swallowing
○ Stomach fullness or bloating ○ Wheezing or dry cough

Other symptoms: _____

Post-dinner energy level: ○ low ○ medium ○ high

Snack

Time: _____

List the foods you ate as a snack.

_____   _____

Drink _____   ○ room-temp ○ hot ○ cold

Comments: _____

Post-snack energy level: ○ low ○ medium ○ high

Snack

Time: _____

List the foods you ate as a snack.

_____   _____

Drink _____   ○ room-temp ○ hot ○ cold

Comments: _____

Post-snack energy level: ○ low ○ medium ○ high

Medications & Supplements

Include prescription medication, over-the-counter medication & vitamin supplements.

_____   _____

_____   _____

_____   _____

_____   _____

_____   _____

Energy level | Restfulness

Today's waking energy level?
○ low   ○ medium   ○ high

# of times roused from sleep last night?
○ 1   ○ 2   ○ 3+

Last night's reflux/GERD symptoms:

_____   _____

_____   _____

Bed raised?   ○ Y   ○ N   Wedged Pillows?   ○ Y   ○ N

Last meal time? _____   Approx bedtime? _____ am pm
(Remember to give yourself at least 2-3 hours after meals before lying down.)

End-of-day notes

Noticeable change in symptoms? _(Ex: "Throat discomfort has completely disappeared.")_

_____

_____

New terms to research   Books & websites with helpful info

_____   _____

_____   _____

Additional notes:

_____

_____

_____

Breakfast   Time: _____

List the foods you ate for breakfast.

_____   _____

_____   _____

_____   _____

Drink _____   **Drink** _____
○ room-temp ○ hot ○ cold   ○ room-temp ○ hot ○ cold

Comments:

Physical symptoms after meal: ○ **low**   ○ **intense**   ○ **non-existent**
○ Belching   ○ Upper abdominal pain and discomfort
○ Nausea   ○ Difficulty or pain with swallowing
○ Stomach fullness or bloating   ○ Wheezing or dry cough

Other symptoms:

Post-breakfast energy level: ○ low   ○ medium   ○ high

Lunch   Time: _____

List the foods you ate for lunch.

_____   _____

_____   _____

_____   _____

Drink _____   **Drink** _____
○ room-temp ○ hot ○ cold   ○ room-temp ○ hot ○ cold

Comments:

Physical symptoms after meal: ○ **low**   ○ **intense**   ○ **non-existent**
○ Belching   ○ Upper abdominal pain and discomfort
○ Nausea   ○ Difficulty or pain with swallowing
○ Stomach fullness or bloating   ○ Wheezing or dry cough

Other symptoms:

Post-lunch energy level: ○ low   ○ medium   ○ high

Dinner

Time: _____

List the foods you ate for dinner.

_____   _____

_____   _____

_____   _____

Drink _____   **Drink** _____
○ room-temp   ○ hot   ○ cold   ○ room-temp   ○ hot   ○ cold

Comments: _____

Physical symptoms after meal: ○ **low**   ○ **intense**   ○ **non-existent**
○ Belching   ○ Upper abdominal pain and discomfort
○ Nausea   ○ Difficulty or pain with swallowing
○ Stomach fullness or bloating   ○ Wheezing or dry cough

Other symptoms: _____

Post-dinner energy level: ○ low   ○ medium   ○ high

Snack

Time: _____

List the foods you ate as a snack.

_____   _____

Drink _____   ○ room-temp   ○ hot   ○ cold

Comments: _____

Post-snack energy level: ○ low   ○ medium   ○ high

Snack

Time: _____

List the foods you ate as a snack.

_____   _____

Drink _____   ○ room-temp   ○ hot   ○ cold

Comments: _____

Post-snack energy level: ○ low   ○ medium   ○ high

Medications & Supplements

Include prescription medication, over-the-counter medication & vitamin supplements.

_____   _____

_____   _____

_____   _____

_____   _____

_____   _____

Energy level | Restfulness

Today's waking energy level?
○ low   ○ medium   ○ high

# of times roused from sleep last night?
○ 1   ○ 2   ○ 3+

Last night's reflux/GERD symptoms:

_____   _____

_____   _____

Bed raised?   ○ Y   ○ N   Wedged Pillows?   ○ Y   ○ N

Last meal time? _____   Approx bedtime? _____   am   pm
(Remember to give yourself at least 2-3 hours after meals before lying down.)

End-of-day notes

Noticeable change in symptoms? _(Ex: "Throat discomfort has completely disappeared.")_

_____

_____

New terms to research   Books & websites with helpful info

_____   _____

_____   _____

Additional notes:

_____

_____

_____

Breakfast

Time: _____

List the foods you ate for breakfast.

_____   _____

_____   _____

_____   _____

Drink _____   **Drink** _____
  ○ room-temp   ○ hot   ○ cold   ○ room-temp   ○ hot   ○ cold

Comments: _____

Physical symptoms after meal: ○ **low**   ○ **intense**   ○ **non-existent**
○ Belching   ○ Upper abdominal pain and discomfort
○ Nausea   ○ Difficulty or pain with swallowing
○ Stomach fullness or bloating   ○ Wheezing or dry cough

Other symptoms: _____

Post-breakfast energy level: ○ low   ○ medium   ○ high

Lunch

Time: _____

List the foods you ate for lunch.

_____   _____

_____   _____

_____   _____

Drink _____   **Drink** _____
  ○ room-temp   ○ hot   ○ cold   ○ room-temp   ○ hot   ○ cold

Comments: _____

Physical symptoms after meal: ○ **low**   ○ **intense**   ○ **non-existent**
○ Belching   ○ Upper abdominal pain and discomfort
○ Nausea   ○ Difficulty or pain with swallowing
○ Stomach fullness or bloating   ○ Wheezing or dry cough

Other symptoms: _____

Post-lunch energy level: ○ low   ○ medium   ○ high

Dinner

Time: _____

List the foods you ate for dinner.

_____   _____

_____   _____

_____   _____

Drink _____   **Drink** _____
○ room-temp   ○ hot   ○ cold   ○ room-temp   ○ hot   ○ cold

Comments:

_____

Physical symptoms after meal: ○ **low**   ○ **intense**   ○ **non-existent**
○ Belching   ○ Upper abdominal pain and discomfort
○ Nausea   ○ Difficulty or pain with swallowing
○ Stomach fullness or bloating   ○ Wheezing or dry cough

Other symptoms:

Post-dinner energy level: ○ low   ○ medium   ○ high

Snack

Time: _____

List the foods you ate as a snack.

_____   _____

Drink _____   ○ room-temp   ○ hot   ○ cold

Comments: _____

Post-snack energy level: ○ low   ○ medium   ○ high

Snack

Time: _____

List the foods you ate as a snack.

_____   _____

Drink _____   ○ room-temp   ○ hot   ○ cold

Comments: _____

Post-snack energy level: ○ low   ○ medium   ○ high

Medications & Supplements

Include prescription medication, over-the-counter medication & vitamin supplements.

_____   _____

_____   _____

_____   _____

_____   _____

_____   _____

Energy level | Restfulness

Today's waking energy level?
○ low   ○ medium   ○ high

# of times roused from sleep last night?
○ 1   ○ 2   ○ 3+

Last night's reflux/GERD symptoms:

_____   _____

_____   _____

Bed raised?   ○ Y   ○ N   Wedged Pillows?   ○ Y   ○ N

Last meal time? _____   Approx bedtime? _____ am pm
(Remember to give yourself at least 2-3 hours after meals before lying down.)

End-of-day notes

Noticeable change in symptoms? _(Ex: "Throat discomfort has completely disappeared.")_

_____

_____

New terms to research   Books & websites with helpful info

_____   _____

_____   _____

Additional notes:

_____

_____

_____

DATE

Breakfast   Time: _____

List the foods you ate for breakfast.

_____   _____

_____   _____

_____   _____

Drink _____   **Drink** _____
○ room-temp ○ hot ○ cold   ○ room-temp ○ hot ○ cold

Comments: _____

Physical symptoms after meal: ○ **low** ○ **intense** ○ **non-existent**
○ Belching   ○ Upper abdominal pain and discomfort
○ Nausea   ○ Difficulty or pain with swallowing
○ Stomach fullness or bloating ○ Wheezing or dry cough

Other symptoms: _____

Post-breakfast energy level: ○ low ○ medium ○ high

Lunch   Time: _____

List the foods you ate for lunch.

_____   _____

_____   _____

_____   _____

Drink _____   **Drink** _____
○ room-temp ○ hot ○ cold   ○ room-temp ○ hot ○ cold

Comments: _____

Physical symptoms after meal: ○ **low** ○ **intense** ○ **non-existent**
○ Belching   ○ Upper abdominal pain and discomfort
○ Nausea   ○ Difficulty or pain with swallowing
○ Stomach fullness or bloating ○ Wheezing or dry cough

Other symptoms: _____

Post-lunch energy level: ○ low ○ medium ○ high

Dinner

Time: _____

List the foods you ate for dinner.

_____   _____

_____   _____

_____   _____

Drink _____   **Drink** _____

  ○ room-temp ○ hot ○ cold   ○ room-temp ○ hot ○ cold

Comments:

Physical symptoms after meal: ○ **low** ○ **intense** ○ **non-existent**

○ Belching   ○ Upper abdominal pain and discomfort

○ Nausea   ○ Difficulty or pain with swallowing

○ Stomach fullness or bloating ○ Wheezing or dry cough

Other symptoms:

Post-dinner energy level: ○ low ○ medium ○ high

Snack

Time: _____

List the foods you ate as a snack.

_____   _____

Drink _____ ○ room-temp ○ hot ○ cold

Comments:

Post-snack energy level: ○ low ○ medium ○ high

Snack

Time: _____

List the foods you ate as a snack.

_____   _____

Drink _____ ○ room-temp ○ hot ○ cold

Comments:

Post-snack energy level: ○ low ○ medium ○ high

Medications & Supplements

Include prescription medication, over-the-counter medication & vitamin supplements.

_____   _____

_____   _____

_____   _____

_____   _____

_____   _____

Energy level | Restfulness

Today's waking energy level?
○ low   ○ medium   ○ high

# of times roused from sleep last night?
○ 1   ○ 2   ○ 3+

Last night's reflux/GERD symptoms:

_____   _____

_____   _____

Bed raised?   ○ Y   ○ N   Wedged Pillows?   ○ Y   ○ N

Last meal time? _____   Approx bedtime? _____ am pm
(Remember to give yourself at least 2-3 hours after meals before lying down.)

End-of-day notes

Noticeable change in symptoms? _(Ex: "Throat discomfort has completely disappeared.")_

_____

_____

New terms to research   Books & websites with helpful info

_____   _____

_____   _____

Additional notes:

_____

_____

_____

Breakfast

Time: _____

List the foods you ate for breakfast.

_____   _____

_____   _____

_____   _____

Drink _____   **Drink** _____
○ room-temp   ○ hot   ○ cold   ○ room-temp   ○ hot   ○ cold

Comments: _____

Physical symptoms after meal: ○ **low**   ○ **intense**   ○ **non-existent**
○ Belching   ○ Upper abdominal pain and discomfort
○ Nausea   ○ Difficulty or pain with swallowing
○ Stomach fullness or bloating   ○ Wheezing or dry cough

Other symptoms: _____

Post-breakfast energy level: ○ low   ○ medium   ○ high

Lunch

Time: _____

List the foods you ate for lunch.

_____   _____

_____   _____

_____   _____

Drink _____   **Drink** _____
○ room-temp   ○ hot   ○ cold   ○ room-temp   ○ hot   ○ cold

Comments: _____

Physical symptoms after meal: ○ **low**   ○ **intense**   ○ **non-existent**
○ Belching   ○ Upper abdominal pain and discomfort
○ Nausea   ○ Difficulty or pain with swallowing
○ Stomach fullness or bloating   ○ Wheezing or dry cough

Other symptoms: _____

Post-lunch energy level: ○ low   ○ medium   ○ high

Dinner

Time: _____

List the foods you ate for dinner.

_____   _____

_____   _____

_____   _____

Drink _____   **Drink** _____
○ room-temp ○ hot ○ cold   ○ room-temp ○ hot ○ cold

Comments: _____

Physical symptoms after meal: ○ **low**   ○ **intense**   ○ **non-existent**
○ Belching   ○ Upper abdominal pain and discomfort
○ Nausea   ○ Difficulty or pain with swallowing
○ Stomach fullness or bloating ○ Wheezing or dry cough

Other symptoms: _____

Post-dinner energy level: ○ low ○ medium ○ high

Snack

Time: _____

List the foods you ate as a snack.

_____   _____

Drink _____   ○ room-temp ○ hot ○ cold

Comments: _____

Post-snack energy level: ○ low ○ medium ○ high

Snack

Time: _____

List the foods you ate as a snack.

_____   _____

Drink _____   ○ room-temp ○ hot ○ cold

Comments: _____

Post-snack energy level: ○ low ○ medium ○ high

Medications & Supplements

Include prescription medication, over-the-counter medication & vitamin supplements.

_____   _____

_____   _____

_____   _____

_____   _____

_____   _____

Energy level | Restfulness

Today's waking energy level?
○ low   ○ medium   ○ high

# of times roused from sleep last night?
○ 1   ○ 2   ○ 3+

Last night's reflux/GERD symptoms:

_____   _____

_____   _____

Bed raised?   ○ Y   ○ N   Wedged Pillows?   ○ Y   ○ N

Last meal time? _____   Approx bedtime? _____ am pm
(Remember to give yourself at least 2-3 hours after meals before lying down.)

End-of-day notes

Noticeable change in symptoms? *(Ex: "Throat discomfort has completely disappeared.")*

_____

_____

New terms to research   Books & websites with helpful info

_____   _____

_____   _____

Additional notes:

_____

_____

_____

Breakfast

Time: _____

List the foods you ate for breakfast.

_____   _____

_____   _____

_____   _____

Drink _____   **Drink** _____
○ room-temp ○ hot ○ cold   ○ room-temp ○ hot ○ cold

Comments: _____

Physical symptoms after meal: ○ **low** ○ **intense** ○ **non-existent**
○ Belching   ○ Upper abdominal pain and discomfort
○ Nausea   ○ Difficulty or pain with swallowing
○ Stomach fullness or bloating   ○ Wheezing or dry cough

Other symptoms: _____

Post-breakfast energy level: ○ low ○ medium ○ high

Lunch

Time: _____

List the foods you ate for lunch.

_____   _____

_____   _____

_____   _____

Drink _____   **Drink** _____
○ room-temp ○ hot ○ cold   ○ room-temp ○ hot ○ cold

Comments: _____

Physical symptoms after meal: ○ **low** ○ **intense** ○ **non-existent**
○ Belching   ○ Upper abdominal pain and discomfort
○ Nausea   ○ Difficulty or pain with swallowing
○ Stomach fullness or bloating   ○ Wheezing or dry cough

Other symptoms: _____

Post-lunch energy level: ○ low ○ medium ○ high

Dinner

Time: _____

List the foods you ate for dinner.

_____   _____

_____   _____

_____   _____

Drink _____   **Drink** _____
    ○ room-temp ○ hot ○ cold   ○ room-temp ○ hot ○ cold

Comments: _____

Physical symptoms after meal: ○ **low** ○ **intense** ○ **non-existent**
○ Belching   ○ Upper abdominal pain and discomfort
○ Nausea   ○ Difficulty or pain with swallowing
○ Stomach fullness or bloating   ○ Wheezing or dry cough

Other symptoms: _____

Post-dinner energy level: ○ low ○ medium ○ high

Snack

Time: _____

List the foods you ate as a snack.

_____   _____

Drink _____   ○ room-temp ○ hot ○ cold

Comments: _____

Post-snack energy level: ○ low ○ medium ○ high

Snack

Time: _____

List the foods you ate as a snack.

_____   _____

Drink _____   ○ room-temp ○ hot ○ cold

Comments: _____

Post-snack energy level: ○ low ○ medium ○ high

Medications & Supplements

Include prescription medication, over-the-counter medication & vitamin supplements.

_____   _____

_____   _____

_____   _____

_____   _____

_____   _____

Energy level | Restfulness

Today's waking energy level?
○ low   ○ medium   ○ high

# of times roused from sleep last night?
○ 1   ○ 2   ○ 3+

Last night's reflux/GERD symptoms:

_____   _____

_____   _____

Bed raised?   ○ Y   ○ N   Wedged Pillows?   ○ Y   ○ N

Last meal time? _____   Approx bedtime? _____   am   pm
(Remember to give yourself at least 2-3 hours after meals before lying down.)

End-of-day notes

Noticeable change in symptoms? *(Ex: "Throat discomfort has completely disappeared.")*

_____

_____

New terms to research   Books & websites with helpful info

_____   _____

_____   _____

Additional notes:

_____

_____

_____

Breakfast   Time: _____

List the foods you ate for breakfast.

_____   _____

_____   _____

_____   _____

Drink _____   **Drink** _____
  ○ room-temp ○ hot ○ cold   ○ room-temp ○ hot ○ cold

Comments: _____

Physical symptoms after meal: ○ **low**   ○ **intense**   ○ **non-existent**
○ Belching   ○ Upper abdominal pain and discomfort
○ Nausea   ○ Difficulty or pain with swallowing
○ Stomach fullness or bloating   ○ Wheezing or dry cough

Other symptoms: _____

Post-breakfast energy level: ○ low   ○ medium   ○ high

Lunch   Time: _____

List the foods you ate for lunch.

_____   _____

_____   _____

_____   _____

Drink _____   **Drink** _____
  ○ room-temp ○ hot ○ cold   ○ room-temp ○ hot ○ cold

Comments: _____

Physical symptoms after meal: ○ **low**   ○ **intense**   ○ **non-existent**
○ Belching   ○ Upper abdominal pain and discomfort
○ Nausea   ○ Difficulty or pain with swallowing
○ Stomach fullness or bloating   ○ Wheezing or dry cough

Other symptoms: _____

Post-lunch energy level: ○ low   ○ medium   ○ high

Dinner

Time: _____

List the foods you ate for dinner.

_____   _____

_____   _____

_____   _____

Drink _____   **Drink** _____
○ room-temp ○ hot ○ cold   ○ room-temp ○ hot ○ cold

Comments: _____

Physical symptoms after meal: ○ **low** ○ **intense** ○ **non-existent**
○ Belching   ○ Upper abdominal pain and discomfort
○ Nausea   ○ Difficulty or pain with swallowing
○ Stomach fullness or bloating   ○ Wheezing or dry cough

Other symptoms: _____

Post-dinner energy level: ○ low   ○ medium   ○ high

Snack

Time: _____

List the foods you ate as a snack.

_____   _____

Drink _____   ○ room-temp   ○ hot   ○ cold

Comments: _____

Post-snack energy level: ○ low   ○ medium   ○ high

Snack

Time: _____

List the foods you ate as a snack.

_____   _____

Drink _____   ○ room-temp   ○ hot   ○ cold

Comments: _____

Post-snack energy level: ○ low   ○ medium   ○ high

Medications & Supplements

Include prescription medication, over-the-counter medication & vitamin supplements.

_____   _____

_____   _____

_____   _____

_____   _____

_____   _____

Energy level | Restfulness

Today's waking energy level?
○ low   ○ medium   ○ high

# of times roused from sleep last night?
○ 1   ○ 2   ○ 3+

Last night's reflux/GERD symptoms:

_____   _____

_____   _____

Bed raised?   ○ Y   ○ N   Wedged Pillows?   ○ Y   ○ N

Last meal time? _____   Approx bedtime? _____ am pm
       (Remember to give yourself at least 2-3 hours after meals before lying down.)

End-of-day notes

Noticeable change in symptoms? _(Ex: "Throat discomfort has completely disappeared.")_

_____

_____

New terms to research   Books & websites with helpful info

_____   _____

_____   _____

Additional notes:

_____

_____

_____

Breakfast

Time: _____

List the foods you ate for breakfast.

_____   _____

_____   _____

_____   _____

Drink _____   **Drink** _____
○ room-temp   ○ hot   ○ cold   ○ room-temp   ○ hot   ○ cold

Comments: _____

Physical symptoms after meal: ○ **low**   ○ **intense**   ○ **non-existent**
○ Belching   ○ Upper abdominal pain and discomfort
○ Nausea   ○ Difficulty or pain with swallowing
○ Stomach fullness or bloating   ○ Wheezing or dry cough

Other symptoms: _____

Post-breakfast energy level: ○ low   ○ medium   ○ high

Lunch

Time: _____

List the foods you ate for lunch.

_____   _____

_____   _____

_____   _____

Drink _____   **Drink** _____
○ room-temp   ○ hot   ○ cold   ○ room-temp   ○ hot   ○ cold

Comments: _____

Physical symptoms after meal: ○ **low**   ○ **intense**   ○ **non-existent**
○ Belching   ○ Upper abdominal pain and discomfort
○ Nausea   ○ Difficulty or pain with swallowing
○ Stomach fullness or bloating   ○ Wheezing or dry cough

Other symptoms: _____

Post-lunch energy level: ○ low   ○ medium   ○ high

Dinner

Time: _____

List the foods you ate for dinner.

_____   _____

_____   _____

_____   _____

Drink _____   **Drink** _____
○ room-temp   ○ hot   ○ cold   ○ room-temp   ○ hot   ○ cold

Comments: _____

Physical symptoms after meal: ○ **low**   ○ **intense**   ○ **non-existent**
○ Belching   ○ Upper abdominal pain and discomfort
○ Nausea   ○ Difficulty or pain with swallowing
○ Stomach fullness or bloating   ○ Wheezing or dry cough

Other symptoms: _____

Post-dinner energy level: ○ low   ○ medium   ○ high

Snack

Time: _____

List the foods you ate as a snack.

_____   _____

Drink _____   ○ room-temp   ○ hot   ○ cold

Comments: _____

Post-snack energy level: ○ low   ○ medium   ○ high

Snack

Time: _____

List the foods you ate as a snack.

_____   _____

Drink _____   ○ room-temp   ○ hot   ○ cold

Comments: _____

Post-snack energy level: ○ low   ○ medium   ○ high

Medications & Supplements

Include prescription medication, over-the-counter medication & vitamin supplements.

_____   _____

_____   _____

_____   _____

_____   _____

_____   _____

Energy level | Restfulness

Today's waking energy level?
○ low   ○ medium   ○ high

# of times roused from sleep last night?
○ 1   ○ 2   ○ 3+

Last night's reflux/GERD symptoms:

_____   _____

_____   _____

Bed raised?   ○ Y   ○ N   Wedged Pillows?   ○ Y   ○ N

Last meal time? _____   Approx bedtime? _____ am pm
(Remember to give yourself at least 2-3 hours after meals before lying down.)

End-of-day notes

Noticeable change in symptoms? _(Ex: "Throat discomfort has completely disappeared.")_

_____

_____

New terms to research   Books & websites with helpful info

_____   _____

_____   _____

Additional notes:

_____

_____

_____

DATE	

Breakfast   Time: _____

List the foods you ate for breakfast.

_____   _____

_____   _____

_____   _____

Drink _____   **Drink** _____
○ room-temp ○ hot ○ cold   ○ room-temp ○ hot ○ cold

Comments:

Physical symptoms after meal: ○ **low** ○ **intense** ○ **non-existent**
○ Belching   ○ Upper abdominal pain and discomfort
○ Nausea   ○ Difficulty or pain with swallowing
○ Stomach fullness or bloating   ○ Wheezing or dry cough

Other symptoms:

Post-breakfast energy level: ○ low ○ medium ○ high

Lunch   Time: _____

List the foods you ate for lunch.

_____   _____

_____   _____

_____   _____

Drink _____   **Drink** _____
○ room-temp ○ hot ○ cold   ○ room-temp ○ hot ○ cold

Comments:

Physical symptoms after meal: ○ **low** ○ **intense** ○ **non-existent**
○ Belching   ○ Upper abdominal pain and discomfort
○ Nausea   ○ Difficulty or pain with swallowing
○ Stomach fullness or bloating   ○ Wheezing or dry cough

Other symptoms:

Post-lunch energy level: ○ low ○ medium ○ high

Dinner
Time: _____

List the foods you ate for dinner.

_____   _____

_____   _____

_____   _____

Drink _____   **Drink** _____
○ room-temp ○ hot ○ cold   ○ room-temp ○ hot ○ cold

Comments: _____

Physical symptoms after meal: ○ **low** ○ **intense** ○ **non-existent**
○ Belching   ○ Upper abdominal pain and discomfort
○ Nausea   ○ Difficulty or pain with swallowing
○ Stomach fullness or bloating ○ Wheezing or dry cough

Other symptoms: _____

Post-dinner energy level: ○ low   ○ medium   ○ high

Snack
Time: _____

List the foods you ate as a snack.

_____   _____

Drink _____   ○ room-temp ○ hot ○ cold

Comments: _____

Post-snack energy level: ○ low   ○ medium   ○ high

Snack
Time: _____

List the foods you ate as a snack.

_____   _____

Drink _____   ○ room-temp ○ hot ○ cold

Comments: _____

Post-snack energy level: ○ low   ○ medium   ○ high

Medications & Supplements

Include prescription medication, over-the-counter medication & vitamin supplements.

_____   _____

_____   _____

_____   _____

_____   _____

_____   _____

Energy level | Restfulness

Today's waking energy level?
○ low   ○ medium   ○ high

# of times roused from sleep last night?
○ 1   ○ 2   ○ 3+

Last night's reflux/GERD symptoms:

_____   _____

_____   _____

Bed raised?   ○ Y   ○ N   Wedged Pillows?   ○ Y   ○ N

Last meal time? _____   Approx bedtime? _____ am pm
(Remember to give yourself at least 2-3 hours after meals before lying down.)

End-of-day notes

Noticeable change in symptoms? *(Ex: "Throat discomfort has completely disappeared.")*

_____

_____

New terms to research   Books & websites with helpful info

_____   _____

_____   _____

Additional notes:

_____

_____

_____

Breakfast

Time: _____

List the foods you ate for breakfast.

_____   _____

_____   _____

_____   _____

Drink _____   **Drink** _____
○ room-temp ○ hot ○ cold   ○ room-temp ○ hot ○ cold

Comments: _____

Physical symptoms after meal: ○ **low**   ○ **intense**   ○ **non-existent**
○ Belching   ○ Upper abdominal pain and discomfort
○ Nausea   ○ Difficulty or pain with swallowing
○ Stomach fullness or bloating   ○ Wheezing or dry cough

Other symptoms: _____

Post-breakfast energy level: ○ low   ○ medium   ○ high

Lunch

Time: _____

List the foods you ate for lunch.

_____   _____

_____   _____

_____   _____

Drink _____   **Drink** _____
○ room-temp ○ hot ○ cold   ○ room-temp ○ hot ○ cold

Comments: _____

Physical symptoms after meal: ○ **low**   ○ **intense**   ○ **non-existent**
○ Belching   ○ Upper abdominal pain and discomfort
○ Nausea   ○ Difficulty or pain with swallowing
○ Stomach fullness or bloating   ○ Wheezing or dry cough

Other symptoms: _____

Post-lunch energy level: ○ low   ○ medium   ○ high

Dinner

Time: _____

List the foods you ate for dinner.

_____   _____

_____   _____

_____   _____

Drink _____   **Drink** _____
   ○ room-temp   ○ hot   ○ cold   ○ room-temp   ○ hot   ○ cold

Comments: _____

Physical symptoms after meal: ○ **low**   ○ **intense**   ○ **non-existent**

○ Belching   ○ Upper abdominal pain and discomfort
○ Nausea   ○ Difficulty or pain with swallowing
○ Stomach fullness or bloating   ○ Wheezing or dry cough

Other symptoms: _____

Post-dinner energy level: ○ low   ○ medium   ○ high

Snack

Time: _____

List the foods you ate as a snack.

_____   _____

Drink _____   ○ room-temp   ○ hot   ○ cold

Comments: _____

Post-snack energy level: ○ low   ○ medium   ○ high

Snack

Time: _____

List the foods you ate as a snack.

_____   _____

Drink _____   ○ room-temp   ○ hot   ○ cold

Comments: _____

Post-snack energy level: ○ low   ○ medium   ○ high

Medications & Supplements

Include prescription medication, over-the-counter medication & vitamin supplements.

_____   _____

_____   _____

_____   _____

_____   _____

_____   _____

Energy level | Restfulness

Today's waking energy level?
○ low   ○ medium   ○ high

# of times roused from sleep last night?
○ 1   ○ 2   ○ 3+

Last night's reflux/GERD symptoms:

_____   _____

_____   _____

Bed raised?   ○ Y   ○ N   Wedged Pillows?   ○ Y   ○ N

Last meal time? _____   Approx bedtime? _____ am pm
(Remember to give yourself at least 2-3 hours after meals before lying down.)

End-of-day notes

Noticeable change in symptoms? *(Ex: "Throat discomfort has completely disappeared.")*

_____

_____

New terms to research   Books & websites with helpful info

_____   _____

_____   _____

Additional notes:

_____

_____

_____

Breakfast

Time: _____

List the foods you ate for breakfast.

_____   _____

_____   _____

_____   _____

Drink _____   **Drink** _____
  ○ room-temp ○ hot ○ cold   ○ room-temp ○ hot ○ cold

Comments: _____

Physical symptoms after meal: ○ **low**   ○ **intense**   ○ **non-existent**
○ Belching   ○ Upper abdominal pain and discomfort
○ Nausea   ○ Difficulty or pain with swallowing
○ Stomach fullness or bloating ○ Wheezing or dry cough

Other symptoms: _____

Post-breakfast energy level: ○ low   ○ medium   ○ high

Lunch

Time: _____

List the foods you ate for lunch.

_____   _____

_____   _____

_____   _____

Drink _____   **Drink** _____
  ○ room-temp ○ hot ○ cold   ○ room-temp ○ hot ○ cold

Comments: _____

Physical symptoms after meal: ○ **low**   ○ **intense**   ○ **non-existent**
○ Belching   ○ Upper abdominal pain and discomfort
○ Nausea   ○ Difficulty or pain with swallowing
○ Stomach fullness or bloating ○ Wheezing or dry cough

Other symptoms: _____

Post-lunch energy level: ○ low   ○ medium   ○ high

Dinner

Time: _____

List the foods you ate for dinner.

_____   _____

_____   _____

_____   _____

Drink _____   **Drink** _____
  ○ room-temp ○ hot ○ cold   ○ room-temp ○ hot ○ cold

Comments:

Physical symptoms after meal: ○ **low**   ○ **intense**   ○ **non-existent**
○ Belching   ○ Upper abdominal pain and discomfort
○ Nausea   ○ Difficulty or pain with swallowing
○ Stomach fullness or bloating   ○ Wheezing or dry cough

Other symptoms:

Post-dinner energy level: ○ low   ○ medium   ○ high

Snack

Time: _____

List the foods you ate as a snack.

_____

Drink _____   ○ room-temp   ○ hot   ○ cold

Comments:

Post-snack energy level: ○ low   ○ medium   ○ high

Snack

Time: _____

List the foods you ate as a snack.

_____

Drink _____   ○ room-temp   ○ hot   ○ cold

Comments:

Post-snack energy level: ○ low   ○ medium   ○ high

Medications & Supplements

Include prescription medication, over-the-counter medication & vitamin supplements.

_____   _____

_____   _____

_____   _____

_____   _____

_____   _____

Energy level | Restfulness

Today's waking energy level?
○ low   ○ medium   ○ high

# of times roused from sleep last night?
○ 1   ○ 2   ○ 3+

Last night's reflux/GERD symptoms:

_____   _____

_____   _____

Bed raised?   ○ Y   ○ N   Wedged Pillows?   ○ Y   ○ N

Last meal time? _____   Approx bedtime? _____ am pm
(Remember to give yourself at least 2-3 hours after meals before lying down.)

End-of-day notes

Noticeable change in symptoms? _(Ex: "Throat discomfort has completely disappeared.")_

_____

_____

New terms to research   Books & websites with helpful info

_____   _____

_____   _____

Additional notes:

_____

_____

_____

Breakfast   Time: _____

List the foods you ate for breakfast.

_____   _____

_____   _____

_____   _____

Drink _____   **Drink** _____
○ room-temp   ○ hot   ○ cold   ○ room-temp   ○ hot   ○ cold

Comments: _____

Physical symptoms after meal: ○ **low**   ○ **intense**   ○ **non-existent**
○ Belching   ○ Upper abdominal pain and discomfort
○ Nausea   ○ Difficulty or pain with swallowing
○ Stomach fullness or bloating   ○ Wheezing or dry cough

Other symptoms: _____

Post-breakfast energy level: ○ low   ○ medium   ○ high

Lunch   Time: _____

List the foods you ate for lunch.

_____   _____

_____   _____

_____   _____

Drink _____   **Drink** _____
○ room-temp   ○ hot   ○ cold   ○ room-temp   ○ hot   ○ cold

Comments: _____

Physical symptoms after meal: ○ **low**   ○ **intense**   ○ **non-existent**
○ Belching   ○ Upper abdominal pain and discomfort
○ Nausea   ○ Difficulty or pain with swallowing
○ Stomach fullness or bloating   ○ Wheezing or dry cough

Other symptoms: _____

Post-lunch energy level: ○ low   ○ medium   ○ high

Dinner

Time: _____

List the foods you ate for dinner.

_____   _____

_____   _____

_____   _____

Drink _____   **Drink** _____
  ○ room-temp ○ hot ○ cold   ○ room-temp ○ hot ○ cold

Comments:

Physical symptoms after meal: ○ **low** ○ **intense** ○ **non-existent**

○ Belching   ○ Upper abdominal pain and discomfort

○ Nausea   ○ Difficulty or pain with swallowing

○ Stomach fullness or bloating   ○ Wheezing or dry cough

Other symptoms:

Post-dinner energy level: ○ low ○ medium ○ high

Snack

Time: _____

List the foods you ate as a snack.

_____   _____

Drink _____ ○ room-temp ○ hot ○ cold

Comments:

Post-snack energy level: ○ low ○ medium ○ high

Snack

Time: _____

List the foods you ate as a snack.

_____   _____

Drink _____ ○ room-temp ○ hot ○ cold

Comments:

Post-snack energy level: ○ low ○ medium ○ high

Medications & Supplements

Include prescription medication, over-the-counter medication & vitamin supplements.

_____   _____

_____   _____

_____   _____

_____   _____

_____   _____

Energy level | Restfulness

Today's waking energy level?
○ low   ○ medium   ○ high

# of times roused from sleep last night?
○ 1   ○ 2   ○ 3+

Last night's reflux/GERD symptoms:

_____   _____

_____   _____

Bed raised?   ○ Y   ○ N   Wedged Pillows?   ○ Y   ○ N

Last meal time? _____   Approx bedtime? _____ am   pm
(Remember to give yourself at least 2-3 hours after meals before lying down.)

End-of-day notes

Noticeable change in symptoms? *(Ex: "Throat discomfort has completely disappeared.")*

_____

_____

New terms to research   Books & websites with helpful info

_____   _____

_____   _____

Additional notes:

_____

_____

_____

Breakfast

Time: _____

List the foods you ate for breakfast.

_____   _____

_____   _____

_____   _____

Drink _____   **Drink** _____
○ room-temp ○ hot ○ cold   ○ room-temp ○ hot ○ cold

Comments: _____

Physical symptoms after meal: ○ **low**   ○ **intense**   ○ **non-existent**
○ Belching   ○ Upper abdominal pain and discomfort
○ Nausea   ○ Difficulty or pain with swallowing
○ Stomach fullness or bloating   ○ Wheezing or dry cough

Other symptoms: _____

Post-breakfast energy level: ○ low   ○ medium   ○ high

Lunch

Time: _____

List the foods you ate for lunch.

_____   _____

_____   _____

_____   _____

Drink _____   **Drink** _____
○ room-temp ○ hot ○ cold   ○ room-temp ○ hot ○ cold

Comments: _____

Physical symptoms after meal: ○ **low**   ○ **intense**   ○ **non-existent**
○ Belching   ○ Upper abdominal pain and discomfort
○ Nausea   ○ Difficulty or pain with swallowing
○ Stomach fullness or bloating   ○ Wheezing or dry cough

Other symptoms: _____

Post-lunch energy level: ○ low   ○ medium   ○ high

Dinner

Time: _____

List the foods you ate for dinner.

_____   _____

_____   _____

_____   _____

Drink _____   **Drink** _____
  ○ room-temp ○ hot ○ cold   ○ room-temp ○ hot ○ cold

Comments: _____

Physical symptoms after meal: ○ **low**   ○ **intense**   ○ **non-existent**
○ Belching   ○ Upper abdominal pain and discomfort
○ Nausea   ○ Difficulty or pain with swallowing
○ Stomach fullness or bloating ○ Wheezing or dry cough

Other symptoms: _____

Post-dinner energy level: ○ low   ○ medium   ○ high

Snack

Time: _____

List the foods you ate as a snack.

_____   _____

Drink _____   ○ room-temp ○ hot ○ cold

Comments: _____

Post-snack energy level: ○ low   ○ medium   ○ high

Snack

Time: _____

List the foods you ate as a snack.

_____   _____

Drink _____   ○ room-temp ○ hot ○ cold

Comments: _____

Post-snack energy level: ○ low   ○ medium   ○ high

Medications & Supplements

Include prescription medication, over-the-counter medication & vitamin supplements.

_____   _____

_____   _____

_____   _____

_____   _____

_____

Energy level | Restfulness

Today's waking energy level?
○ low   ○ medium   ○ high

# of times roused from sleep last night?
○ 1   ○ 2   ○ 3+

Last night's reflux/GERD symptoms:

_____   _____

_____   _____

Bed raised?   ○ Y   ○ N   Wedged Pillows?   ○ Y   ○ N

Last meal time? _____   Approx bedtime? _____ am pm
(Remember to give yourself at least 2-3 hours after meals before lying down.)

End-of-day notes

Noticeable change in symptoms? _(Ex: "Throat discomfort has completely disappeared.")_

_____

_____

New terms to research   Books & websites with helpful info

_____   _____

_____   _____

Additional notes:

_____

_____

_____

Breakfast   Time: _____

List the foods you ate for breakfast.

_____   _____

_____   _____

_____   _____

Drink _____   **Drink** _____
○ room-temp   ○ hot   ○ cold   ○ room-temp   ○ hot   ○ cold

Comments:

Physical symptoms after meal: ○ **low**   ○ **intense**   ○ **non-existent**
○ Belching   ○ Upper abdominal pain and discomfort
○ Nausea   ○ Difficulty or pain with swallowing
○ Stomach fullness or bloating   ○ Wheezing or dry cough

Other symptoms:

Post-breakfast energy level: ○ low   ○ medium   ○ high

Lunch   Time: _____

List the foods you ate for lunch.

_____   _____

_____   _____

_____   _____

Drink _____   **Drink** _____
○ room-temp   ○ hot   ○ cold   ○ room-temp   ○ hot   ○ cold

Comments:

Physical symptoms after meal: ○ **low**   ○ **intense**   ○ **non-existent**
○ Belching   ○ Upper abdominal pain and discomfort
○ Nausea   ○ Difficulty or pain with swallowing
○ Stomach fullness or bloating   ○ Wheezing or dry cough

Other symptoms:

Post-lunch energy level: ○ low   ○ medium   ○ high

Dinner

Time: _____

List the foods you ate for dinner.

_____   _____

_____   _____

_____   _____

Drink _____   **Drink** _____
○ room-temp   ○ hot   ○ cold   ○ room-temp   ○ hot   ○ cold

Comments:

Physical symptoms after meal: ○ **low**   ○ **intense**   ○ **non-existent**
○ Belching   ○ Upper abdominal pain and discomfort
○ Nausea   ○ Difficulty or pain with swallowing
○ Stomach fullness or bloating   ○ Wheezing or dry cough

Other symptoms:

Post-dinner energy level: ○ low   ○ medium   ○ high

Snack

Time: _____

List the foods you ate as a snack.

_____   _____

Drink _____   ○ room-temp   ○ hot   ○ cold

Comments:

Post-snack energy level: ○ low   ○ medium   ○ high

Snack

Time: _____

List the foods you ate as a snack.

_____   _____

Drink _____   ○ room-temp   ○ hot   ○ cold

Comments:

Post-snack energy level: ○ low   ○ medium   ○ high

Medications & Supplements

Include prescription medication, over-the-counter medication & vitamin supplements.

Energy level | Restfulness

Today's waking energy level?
○ low ○ medium ○ high

# of times roused from sleep last night?
○ 1 ○ 2 ○ 3+

Last night's reflux/GERD symptoms:

_____   _____

_____   _____

Bed raised? ○ Y ○ N   Wedged Pillows? ○ Y ○ N

Last meal time? _____   Approx bedtime? _____ am pm
(Remember to give yourself at least 2-3 hours after meals before lying down.)

End-of-day notes

Noticeable change in symptoms? *(Ex: "Throat discomfort has completely disappeared.")*

_____

_____

New terms to research   Books & websites with helpful info

_____   _____

_____   _____

Additional notes:

_____

_____

_____

Breakfast
Time: _____

List the foods you ate for breakfast.

_____   _____

_____   _____

_____   _____

Drink _____   **Drink** _____
○ room-temp ○ hot ○ cold   ○ room-temp ○ hot ○ cold

Comments: _____

Physical symptoms after meal: ○ **low** ○ **intense** ○ **non-existent**
○ Belching   ○ Upper abdominal pain and discomfort
○ Nausea   ○ Difficulty or pain with swallowing
○ Stomach fullness or bloating ○ Wheezing or dry cough

Other symptoms: _____

Post-breakfast energy level: ○ low ○ medium ○ high

Lunch
Time: _____

List the foods you ate for lunch.

_____   _____

_____   _____

_____   _____

Drink _____   **Drink** _____
○ room-temp ○ hot ○ cold   ○ room-temp ○ hot ○ cold

Comments: _____

Physical symptoms after meal: ○ **low** ○ **intense** ○ **non-existent**
○ Belching   ○ Upper abdominal pain and discomfort
○ Nausea   ○ Difficulty or pain with swallowing
○ Stomach fullness or bloating ○ Wheezing or dry cough

Other symptoms: _____

Post-lunch energy level: ○ low ○ medium ○ high

Dinner

Time: _____

List the foods you ate for dinner.

_____   _____

_____   _____

_____   _____

Drink _____   **Drink** _____
○ room-temp ○ hot ○ cold   ○ room-temp ○ hot ○ cold

Comments:
_____

Physical symptoms after meal: ○ **low** ○ **intense** ○ **non-existent**
○ Belching   ○ Upper abdominal pain and discomfort
○ Nausea   ○ Difficulty or pain with swallowing
○ Stomach fullness or bloating ○ Wheezing or dry cough

Other symptoms:
_____

Post-dinner energy level: ○ low ○ medium ○ high

Snack

Time: _____

List the foods you ate as a snack.

_____   _____

Drink _____   ○ room-temp ○ hot ○ cold

Comments: _____

Post-snack energy level: ○ low ○ medium ○ high

Snack

Time: _____

List the foods you ate as a snack.

_____   _____

Drink _____   ○ room-temp ○ hot ○ cold

Comments: _____

Post-snack energy level: ○ low ○ medium ○ high

Medications & Supplements

Include prescription medication, over-the-counter medication & vitamin supplements.

_____   _____

_____   _____

_____   _____

_____   _____

_____   _____

Energy level | Restfulness

Today's waking energy level?
○ low   ○ medium   ○ high

# of times roused from sleep last night?
○ 1   ○ 2   ○ 3+

Last night's reflux/GERD symptoms:

_____   _____

_____   _____

Bed raised?   ○ Y   ○ N   Wedged Pillows?   ○ Y   ○ N

Last meal time? _____   Approx bedtime? _____ am   pm
(Remember to give yourself at least 2-3 hours after meals before lying down.)

End-of-day notes

Noticeable change in symptoms? *(Ex: "Throat discomfort has completely disappeared.")*

_____

_____

New terms to research   Books & websites with helpful info

_____   _____

_____   _____

Additional notes:

_____

_____

_____

Breakfast   Time: _____

List the foods you ate for breakfast.

_____   _____

_____   _____

_____   _____

Drink _____   **Drink** _____
○ room-temp ○ hot ○ cold   ○ room-temp ○ hot ○ cold

Comments: _____

Physical symptoms after meal: ○ **low** ○ **intense** ○ **non-existent**
○ Belching   ○ Upper abdominal pain and discomfort
○ Nausea   ○ Difficulty or pain with swallowing
○ Stomach fullness or bloating   ○ Wheezing or dry cough

Other symptoms: _____

Post-breakfast energy level: ○ low   ○ medium   ○ high

Lunch   Time: _____

List the foods you ate for lunch.

_____   _____

_____   _____

_____   _____

Drink _____   **Drink** _____
○ room-temp ○ hot ○ cold   ○ room-temp ○ hot ○ cold

Comments: _____

Physical symptoms after meal: ○ **low** ○ **intense** ○ **non-existent**
○ Belching   ○ Upper abdominal pain and discomfort
○ Nausea   ○ Difficulty or pain with swallowing
○ Stomach fullness or bloating   ○ Wheezing or dry cough

Other symptoms: _____

Post-lunch energy level: ○ low   ○ medium   ○ high

Dinner

Time: _____

List the foods you ate for dinner.

_____   _____

_____   _____

_____

Drink _____   **Drink** _____
   ○ room-temp   ○ hot   ○ cold   ○ room-temp   ○ hot   ○ cold

Comments: _____

Physical symptoms after meal: ○ **low**   ○ **intense**   ○ **non-existent**
○ Belching   ○ Upper abdominal pain and discomfort
○ Nausea   ○ Difficulty or pain with swallowing
○ Stomach fullness or bloating   ○ Wheezing or dry cough

Other symptoms: _____

Post-dinner energy level: ○ low   ○ medium   ○ high

Snack

Time: _____

List the foods you ate as a snack.

_____   _____

Drink _____   ○ room-temp   ○ hot   ○ cold

Comments: _____

Post-snack energy level: ○ low   ○ medium   ○ high

Snack

Time: _____

List the foods you ate as a snack.

_____   _____

Drink _____   ○ room-temp   ○ hot   ○ cold

Comments: _____

Post-snack energy level: ○ low   ○ medium   ○ high

Medications & Supplements

Include prescription medication, over-the-counter medication & vitamin supplements.

_____   _____

_____   _____

_____   _____

_____   _____

_____   _____

Energy level | Restfulness

Today's waking energy level?
○ low   ○ medium   ○ high

# of times roused from sleep last night?
○ 1   ○ 2   ○ 3+

Last night's reflux/GERD symptoms:

_____   _____

_____   _____

Bed raised?   ○ Y   ○ N   Wedged Pillows?   ○ Y   ○ N

Last meal time? _____   Approx bedtime? _____ am pm
(Remember to give yourself at least 2-3 hours after meals before lying down.)

End-of-day notes

Noticeable change in symptoms? *(Ex: "Throat discomfort has completely disappeared.")*

_____

_____

New terms to research   Books & websites with helpful info

_____   _____

_____   _____

Additional notes:

_____

_____

_____

Breakfast
Time: _____

List the foods you ate for breakfast.

_____   _____

_____   _____

_____   _____

Drink _____   **Drink** _____
○ room-temp ○ hot ○ cold   ○ room-temp ○ hot ○ cold

Comments: _____

Physical symptoms after meal: ○ **low** ○ **intense** ○ **non-existent**
○ Belching   ○ Upper abdominal pain and discomfort
○ Nausea   ○ Difficulty or pain with swallowing
○ Stomach fullness or bloating ○ Wheezing or dry cough

Other symptoms: _____

Post-breakfast energy level: ○ low ○ medium ○ high

Lunch
Time: _____

List the foods you ate for lunch.

_____   _____

_____   _____

_____   _____

Drink _____   **Drink** _____
○ room-temp ○ hot ○ cold   ○ room-temp ○ hot ○ cold

Comments: _____

Physical symptoms after meal: ○ **low** ○ **intense** ○ **non-existent**
○ Belching   ○ Upper abdominal pain and discomfort
○ Nausea   ○ Difficulty or pain with swallowing
○ Stomach fullness or bloating ○ Wheezing or dry cough

Other symptoms: _____

Post-lunch energy level: ○ low ○ medium ○ high

Dinner

Time: _____

List the foods you ate for dinner.

_____   _____

_____   _____

_____   _____

Drink _____   **Drink** _____
○ room-temp ○ hot ○ cold   ○ room-temp ○ hot ○ cold

Comments: _____

Physical symptoms after meal: ○ **low** ○ **intense** ○ **non-existent**
○ Belching   ○ Upper abdominal pain and discomfort
○ Nausea   ○ Difficulty or pain with swallowing
○ Stomach fullness or bloating ○ Wheezing or dry cough

Other symptoms: _____

Post-dinner energy level: ○ low ○ medium ○ high

Snack

Time: _____

List the foods you ate as a snack.

_____   _____

Drink _____   ○ room-temp ○ hot ○ cold

Comments: _____

Post-snack energy level: ○ low ○ medium ○ high

Snack

Time: _____

List the foods you ate as a snack.

_____   _____

Drink _____   ○ room-temp ○ hot ○ cold

Comments: _____

Post-snack energy level: ○ low ○ medium ○ high

Medications & Supplements

Include prescription medication, over-the-counter medication & vitamin supplements.

_____   _____

_____   _____

_____   _____

_____   _____

_____   _____

Energy level | Restfulness

Today's waking energy level?
○ low   ○ medium   ○ high

# of times roused from sleep last night?
○ 1   ○ 2   ○ 3+

Last night's reflux/GERD symptoms:

_____   _____

_____   _____

Bed raised?   ○ Y   ○ N   Wedged Pillows?   ○ Y   ○ N

Last meal time? _____   Approx bedtime? _____ am pm
(Remember to give yourself at least 2-3 hours after meals before lying down.)

End-of-day notes

Noticeable change in symptoms? _(Ex: "Throat discomfort has completely disappeared.")_

_____

_____

New terms to research   Books & websites with helpful info

_____   _____

_____   _____

Additional notes:

_____

_____

_____

Breakfast

Time: _____

List the foods you ate for breakfast.

_____   _____

_____   _____

_____   _____

Drink _____   **Drink** _____
○ room-temp   ○ hot   ○ cold   ○ room-temp   ○ hot   ○ cold

Comments: _____

Physical symptoms after meal: ○ **low**   ○ **intense**   ○ **non-existent**
○ Belching   ○ Upper abdominal pain and discomfort
○ Nausea   ○ Difficulty or pain with swallowing
○ Stomach fullness or bloating   ○ Wheezing or dry cough

Other symptoms: _____

Post-breakfast energy level: ○ low   ○ medium   ○ high

Lunch

Time: _____

List the foods you ate for lunch.

_____   _____

_____   _____

_____   _____

Drink _____   **Drink** _____
○ room-temp   ○ hot   ○ cold   ○ room-temp   ○ hot   ○ cold

Comments: _____

Physical symptoms after meal: ○ **low**   ○ **intense**   ○ **non-existent**
○ Belching   ○ Upper abdominal pain and discomfort
○ Nausea   ○ Difficulty or pain with swallowing
○ Stomach fullness or bloating   ○ Wheezing or dry cough

Other symptoms: _____

Post-lunch energy level: ○ low   ○ medium   ○ high

Dinner

Time: _____

List the foods you ate for dinner.

_____   _____

_____   _____

_____   _____

Drink _____   **Drink** _____
    ○ room-temp ○ hot ○ cold   ○ room-temp ○ hot ○ cold

Comments:

Physical symptoms after meal: ○ **low**   ○ **intense**   ○ **non-existent**
○ Belching   ○ Upper abdominal pain and discomfort
○ Nausea   ○ Difficulty or pain with swallowing
○ Stomach fullness or bloating   ○ Wheezing or dry cough

Other symptoms: _____

Post-dinner energy level: ○ low ○ medium ○ high

Snack

Time: _____

List the foods you ate as a snack.

_____   _____

Drink _____   ○ room-temp ○ hot ○ cold

Comments: _____

Post-snack energy level: ○ low ○ medium ○ high

Snack

Time: _____

List the foods you ate as a snack.

_____   _____

Drink _____   ○ room-temp ○ hot ○ cold

Comments: _____

Post-snack energy level: ○ low ○ medium ○ high

Medications & Supplements

Include prescription medication, over-the-counter medication & vitamin supplements.

_____   _____

_____   _____

_____   _____

_____   _____

_____   _____

Energy level | Restfulness

Today's waking energy level?
○ low   ○ medium   ○ high

# of times roused from sleep last night?
○ 1   ○ 2   ○ 3+

Last night's reflux/GERD symptoms:

_____   _____

_____   _____

Bed raised?   ○ Y   ○ N   Wedged Pillows?   ○ Y   ○ N

Last meal time? _____   Approx bedtime? _____ am pm
(Remember to give yourself at least 2-3 hours after meals before lying down.)

End-of-day notes

Noticeable change in symptoms? _(Ex: "Throat discomfort has completely disappeared.")_

_____

_____

New terms to research   Books & websites with helpful info

_____   _____

_____   _____

Additional notes:

_____

_____

_____

Breakfast

Time: _____

List the foods you ate for breakfast.

_____   _____

_____   _____

_____   _____

Drink _____   **Drink** _____
   ○ room-temp ○ hot ○ cold   ○ room-temp ○ hot ○ cold

Comments: _____

Physical symptoms after meal: ○ **low**   ○ **intense**   ○ **non-existent**
○ Belching   ○ Upper abdominal pain and discomfort
○ Nausea   ○ Difficulty or pain with swallowing
○ Stomach fullness or bloating ○ Wheezing or dry cough

Other symptoms: _____

Post-breakfast energy level: ○ low   ○ medium   ○ high

Lunch

Time: _____

List the foods you ate for lunch.

_____   _____

_____   _____

_____   _____

Drink _____   **Drink** _____
   ○ room-temp ○ hot ○ cold   ○ room-temp ○ hot ○ cold

Comments: _____

Physical symptoms after meal: ○ **low**   ○ **intense**   ○ **non-existent**
○ Belching   ○ Upper abdominal pain and discomfort
○ Nausea   ○ Difficulty or pain with swallowing
○ Stomach fullness or bloating ○ Wheezing or dry cough

Other symptoms: _____

Post-lunch energy level: ○ low   ○ medium   ○ high

Dinner

Time: _____

List the foods you ate for dinner.

_____   _____

_____   _____

_____   _____

Drink _____ **Drink** _____
○ room-temp ○ hot ○ cold   ○ room-temp ○ hot ○ cold

Comments: _____

Physical symptoms after meal: ○ **low**   ○ **intense**   ○ **non-existent**
○ Belching   ○ Upper abdominal pain and discomfort
○ Nausea   ○ Difficulty or pain with swallowing
○ Stomach fullness or bloating ○ Wheezing or dry cough

Other symptoms: _____

Post-dinner energy level: ○ low   ○ medium   ○ high

Snack

Time: _____

List the foods you ate as a snack.

_____   _____

Drink _____   ○ room-temp   ○ hot   ○ cold

Comments: _____

Post-snack energy level: ○ low   ○ medium   ○ high

Snack

Time: _____

List the foods you ate as a snack.

_____   _____

Drink _____   ○ room-temp   ○ hot   ○ cold

Comments: _____

Post-snack energy level: ○ low   ○ medium   ○ high

Medications & Supplements

Include prescription medication, over-the-counter medication & vitamin supplements.

_____   _____

_____   _____

_____   _____

_____   _____

_____   _____

Energy level | Restfulness

Today's waking energy level?
○ low   ○ medium   ○ high

# of times roused from sleep last night?
○ 1   ○ 2   ○ 3+

Last night's reflux/GERD symptoms:

_____   _____

_____   _____

Bed raised?   ○ Y   ○ N   Wedged Pillows?   ○ Y   ○ N

Last meal time? _____   Approx bedtime? _____ am pm
(Remember to give yourself at least 2-3 hours after meals before lying down.)

End-of-day notes

Noticeable change in symptoms? *(Ex: "Throat discomfort has completely disappeared.")*

_____

_____

New terms to research   Books & websites with helpful info

_____   _____

_____   _____

Additional notes:

_____

_____

_____

Breakfast

Time: _____

List the foods you ate for breakfast.

_____   _____

_____   _____

_____   _____

Drink _____   **Drink** _____
○ room-temp ○ hot ○ cold   ○ room-temp ○ hot ○ cold

Comments: _____

Physical symptoms after meal: ○ **low** ○ **intense** ○ **non-existent**
○ Belching   ○ Upper abdominal pain and discomfort
○ Nausea   ○ Difficulty or pain with swallowing
○ Stomach fullness or bloating   ○ Wheezing or dry cough

Other symptoms: _____

Post-breakfast energy level: ○ low ○ medium ○ high

Lunch

Time: _____

List the foods you ate for lunch.

_____   _____

_____   _____

_____   _____

Drink _____   **Drink** _____
○ room-temp ○ hot ○ cold   ○ room-temp ○ hot ○ cold

Comments: _____

Physical symptoms after meal: ○ **low** ○ **intense** ○ **non-existent**
○ Belching   ○ Upper abdominal pain and discomfort
○ Nausea   ○ Difficulty or pain with swallowing
○ Stomach fullness or bloating   ○ Wheezing or dry cough

Other symptoms: _____

Post-lunch energy level: ○ low ○ medium ○ high

Dinner

Time: _____

List the foods you ate for dinner.

_____   _____

_____   _____

_____   _____

Drink _____
- ○ room-temp ○ hot ○ cold

Drink _____
- ○ room-temp ○ hot ○ cold

Comments: _____

Physical symptoms after meal: ○ **low** ○ **intense** ○ **non-existent**
- ○ Belching
- ○ Nausea
- ○ Stomach fullness or bloating
- ○ Upper abdominal pain and discomfort
- ○ Difficulty or pain with swallowing
- ○ Wheezing or dry cough

Other symptoms: _____

Post-dinner energy level: ○ low ○ medium ○ high

Snack

Time: _____

List the foods you ate as a snack.

_____   _____

Drink _____   ○ room-temp ○ hot ○ cold

Comments: _____

Post-snack energy level: ○ low ○ medium ○ high

Snack

Time: _____

List the foods you ate as a snack.

_____   _____

Drink _____   ○ room-temp ○ hot ○ cold

Comments: _____

Post-snack energy level: ○ low ○ medium ○ high

Medications & Supplements

Include prescription medication, over-the-counter medication & vitamin supplements.

_____   _____

_____   _____

_____   _____

_____   _____

_____   _____

Energy level | Restfulness

Today's waking energy level?
○ low   ○ medium   ○ high

# of times roused from sleep last night?
○ 1   ○ 2   ○ 3+

Last night's reflux/GERD symptoms:

_____   _____

_____   _____

Bed raised?   ○ Y   ○ N   Wedged Pillows?   ○ Y   ○ N

Last meal time? _____   Approx bedtime? _____   am   pm
(Remember to give yourself at least 2-3 hours after meals before lying down.)

End-of-day notes

Noticeable change in symptoms? _(Ex: "Throat discomfort has completely disappeared.")_

_____

_____

New terms to research   Books & websites with helpful info

_____   _____

_____   _____

Additional notes:

_____

_____

_____

Breakfast   Time: _____

List the foods you ate for breakfast.

_____   _____

_____   _____

_____   _____

Drink _____   **Drink** _____
  ○ room-temp   ○ hot   ○ cold   ○ room-temp   ○ hot   ○ cold

Comments: _____

Physical symptoms after meal: ○ **low**   ○ **intense**   ○ **non-existent**
○ Belching   ○ Upper abdominal pain and discomfort
○ Nausea   ○ Difficulty or pain with swallowing
○ Stomach fullness or bloating   ○ Wheezing or dry cough

Other symptoms: _____

Post-breakfast energy level: ○ low   ○ medium   ○ high

Lunch   Time: _____

List the foods you ate for lunch.

_____   _____

_____   _____

_____   _____

Drink _____   **Drink** _____
  ○ room-temp   ○ hot   ○ cold   ○ room-temp   ○ hot   ○ cold

Comments: _____

Physical symptoms after meal: ○ **low**   ○ **intense**   ○ **non-existent**
○ Belching   ○ Upper abdominal pain and discomfort
○ Nausea   ○ Difficulty or pain with swallowing
○ Stomach fullness or bloating   ○ Wheezing or dry cough

Other symptoms: _____

Post-lunch energy level: ○ low   ○ medium   ○ high

Dinner

Time: _____

List the foods you ate for dinner.

_____   _____

_____   _____

_____   _____

Drink _____   **Drink** _____
  ○ room-temp   ○ hot   ○ cold   ○ room-temp   ○ hot   ○ cold

Comments: _____

Physical symptoms after meal: ○ **low**   ○ **intense**   ○ **non-existent**
  ○ Belching   ○ Upper abdominal pain and discomfort
  ○ Nausea   ○ Difficulty or pain with swallowing
  ○ Stomach fullness or bloating   ○ Wheezing or dry cough

Other symptoms: _____

Post-dinner energy level: ○ low   ○ medium   ○ high

Snack

Time: _____

List the foods you ate as a snack.

_____   _____

Drink _____   ○ room-temp   ○ hot   ○ cold

Comments: _____

Post-snack energy level: ○ low   ○ medium   ○ high

Snack

Time: _____

List the foods you ate as a snack.

_____   _____

Drink _____   ○ room-temp   ○ hot   ○ cold

Comments: _____

Post-snack energy level: ○ low   ○ medium   ○ high

Medications & Supplements

Include prescription medication, over-the-counter medication & vitamin supplements.

_____   _____

_____   _____

_____   _____

_____   _____

_____   _____

Energy level | Restfulness

Today's waking energy level?
○ low   ○ medium   ○ high

# of times roused from sleep last night?
○ 1   ○ 2   ○ 3+

Last night's reflux/GERD symptoms:

_____   _____

_____   _____

Bed raised?   ○ Y   ○ N   Wedged Pillows?   ○ Y   ○ N

Last meal time? _____   Approx bedtime? _____ am   pm
(Remember to give yourself at least 2-3 hours after meals before lying down.)

End-of-day notes

Noticeable change in symptoms? *(Ex: "Throat discomfort has completely disappeared.")*

_____

_____

New terms to research   Books & websites with helpful info

_____   _____

_____   _____

Additional notes:

_____

_____

_____

DATE	

Breakfast   Time: _____

List the foods you ate for breakfast.

_____   _____

_____   _____

_____   _____

Drink _____   **Drink** _____
○ room-temp ○ hot ○ cold   ○ room-temp ○ hot ○ cold

Comments: _____

Physical symptoms after meal: ○ **low**   ○ **intense**   ○ **non-existent**
○ Belching   ○ Upper abdominal pain and discomfort
○ Nausea   ○ Difficulty or pain with swallowing
○ Stomach fullness or bloating   ○ Wheezing or dry cough

Other symptoms: _____

Post-breakfast energy level: ○ low   ○ medium   ○ high

Lunch   Time: _____

List the foods you ate for lunch.

_____   _____

_____   _____

_____   _____

Drink _____   **Drink** _____
○ room-temp ○ hot ○ cold   ○ room-temp ○ hot ○ cold

Comments: _____

Physical symptoms after meal: ○ **low**   ○ **intense**   ○ **non-existent**
○ Belching   ○ Upper abdominal pain and discomfort
○ Nausea   ○ Difficulty or pain with swallowing
○ Stomach fullness or bloating   ○ Wheezing or dry cough

Other symptoms: _____

Post-lunch energy level: ○ low   ○ medium   ○ high

Dinner

Time: _____

List the foods you ate for dinner.

_____   _____

_____   _____

_____   _____

Drink _____   **Drink** _____
○ room-temp   ○ hot   ○ cold   ○ room-temp   ○ hot   ○ cold

Comments: _____

Physical symptoms after meal: ○ **low**   ○ **intense**   ○ **non-existent**
○ Belching   ○ Upper abdominal pain and discomfort
○ Nausea   ○ Difficulty or pain with swallowing
○ Stomach fullness or bloating   ○ Wheezing or dry cough

Other symptoms: _____

Post-dinner energy level: ○ low   ○ medium   ○ high

Snack

Time: _____

List the foods you ate as a snack.

_____   _____

Drink _____   ○ room-temp   ○ hot   ○ cold

Comments: _____

Post-snack energy level: ○ low   ○ medium   ○ high

Snack

Time: _____

List the foods you ate as a snack.

_____   _____

Drink _____   ○ room-temp   ○ hot   ○ cold

Comments: _____

Post-snack energy level: ○ low   ○ medium   ○ high

Medications & Supplements

Include prescription medication, over-the-counter medication & vitamin supplements.

_____   _____

_____   _____

_____   _____

_____   _____

_____   _____

Energy level | Restfulness

Today's waking energy level?
○ low   ○ medium   ○ high

# of times roused from sleep last night?
○ 1   ○ 2   ○ 3+

Last night's reflux/GERD symptoms:

_____   _____

_____   _____

Bed raised?   ○ Y   ○ N   Wedged Pillows?   ○ Y   ○ N

Last meal time? _____   Approx bedtime? _____   am   pm
(Remember to give yourself at least 2-3 hours after meals before lying down.)

End-of-day notes

Noticeable change in symptoms? *(Ex: "Throat discomfort has completely disappeared.")*

_____

_____

New terms to research   Books & websites with helpful info

_____   _____

_____   _____

Additional notes:

_____

_____

_____

Breakfast
Time: _____

List the foods you ate for breakfast.

_____   _____

_____   _____

_____   _____

Drink _____   **Drink** _____
○ room-temp ○ hot ○ cold   ○ room-temp ○ hot ○ cold

Comments:
_____

Physical symptoms after meal: ○ **low**   ○ **intense**   ○ **non-existent**
○ Belching   ○ Upper abdominal pain and discomfort
○ Nausea   ○ Difficulty or pain with swallowing
○ Stomach fullness or bloating   ○ Wheezing or dry cough

Other symptoms:
_____

Post-breakfast energy level: ○ low   ○ medium   ○ high

Lunch
Time: _____

List the foods you ate for lunch.

_____   _____

_____   _____

_____   _____

Drink _____   **Drink** _____
○ room-temp ○ hot ○ cold   ○ room-temp ○ hot ○ cold

Comments:
_____

Physical symptoms after meal: ○ **low**   ○ **intense**   ○ **non-existent**
○ Belching   ○ Upper abdominal pain and discomfort
○ Nausea   ○ Difficulty or pain with swallowing
○ Stomach fullness or bloating   ○ Wheezing or dry cough

Other symptoms:
_____

Post-lunch energy level: ○ low   ○ medium   ○ high

Dinner

Time: _____

List the foods you ate for dinner.

_____   _____

_____   _____

_____   _____

Drink _____   **Drink** _____
○ room-temp   ○ hot   ○ cold   ○ room-temp   ○ hot   ○ cold

Comments: _____

Physical symptoms after meal: ○ **low**   ○ **intense**   ○ **non-existent**
○ Belching   ○ Upper abdominal pain and discomfort
○ Nausea   ○ Difficulty or pain with swallowing
○ Stomach fullness or bloating   ○ Wheezing or dry cough

Other symptoms: _____

Post-dinner energy level: ○ low   ○ medium   ○ high

Snack

Time: _____

List the foods you ate as a snack.

_____   _____

Drink _____   ○ room-temp   ○ hot   ○ cold

Comments: _____

Post-snack energy level: ○ low   ○ medium   ○ high

Snack

Time: _____

List the foods you ate as a snack.

_____   _____

Drink _____   ○ room-temp   ○ hot   ○ cold

Comments: _____

Post-snack energy level: ○ low   ○ medium   ○ high

Medications & Supplements

Include prescription medication, over-the-counter medication & vitamin supplements.

_____   _____

_____   _____

_____   _____

_____   _____

_____   _____

Energy level | Restfulness

Today's waking energy level?
○ low   ○ medium   ○ high

# of times roused from sleep last night?
○ 1   ○ 2   ○ 3+

Last night's reflux/GERD symptoms:

_____   _____

_____   _____

Bed raised?   ○ Y   ○ N   Wedged Pillows?   ○ Y   ○ N

Last meal time? _____   Approx bedtime? _____ am pm
(Remember to give yourself at least 2-3 hours after meals before lying down.)

End-of-day notes

Noticeable change in symptoms? _(Ex: "Throat discomfort has completely disappeared.")_

_____

_____

New terms to research   Books & websites with helpful info

_____   _____

_____   _____

Additional notes:

_____

_____

_____

Breakfast
Time: _____

List the foods you ate for breakfast.

_____   _____

_____   _____

_____   _____

Drink _____   **Drink** _____
○ room-temp ○ hot ○ cold   ○ room-temp ○ hot ○ cold

Comments:

Physical symptoms after meal: ○ **low** ○ **intense** ○ **non-existent**
○ Belching   ○ Upper abdominal pain and discomfort
○ Nausea   ○ Difficulty or pain with swallowing
○ Stomach fullness or bloating ○ Wheezing or dry cough

Other symptoms:

Post-breakfast energy level: ○ low   ○ medium   ○ high

Lunch
Time: _____

List the foods you ate for lunch.

_____   _____

_____   _____

_____   _____

Drink _____   **Drink** _____
○ room-temp ○ hot ○ cold   ○ room-temp ○ hot ○ cold

Comments:

Physical symptoms after meal: ○ **low** ○ **intense** ○ **non-existent**
○ Belching   ○ Upper abdominal pain and discomfort
○ Nausea   ○ Difficulty or pain with swallowing
○ Stomach fullness or bloating ○ Wheezing or dry cough

Other symptoms:

Post-lunch energy level: ○ low   ○ medium   ○ high

Dinner

Time: _____

List the foods you ate for dinner.

_____   _____

_____   _____

_____   _____

Drink _____   **Drink** _____
○ room-temp ○ hot ○ cold   ○ room-temp ○ hot ○ cold

Comments: _____

Physical symptoms after meal: ○ **low**   ○ **intense**   ○ **non-existent**
○ Belching   ○ Upper abdominal pain and discomfort
○ Nausea   ○ Difficulty or pain with swallowing
○ Stomach fullness or bloating ○ Wheezing or dry cough

Other symptoms: _____

Post-dinner energy level: ○ low   ○ medium   ○ high

Snack

Time: _____

List the foods you ate as a snack.

_____   _____

Drink _____   ○ room-temp ○ hot ○ cold

Comments: _____

Post-snack energy level: ○ low   ○ medium   ○ high

Snack

Time: _____

List the foods you ate as a snack.

_____   _____

Drink _____   ○ room-temp ○ hot ○ cold

Comments: _____

Post-snack energy level: ○ low   ○ medium   ○ high

Medications & Supplements

Include prescription medication, over-the-counter medication & vitamin supplements.

_____   _____

_____   _____

_____   _____

_____   _____

_____   _____

Energy level | Restfulness

Today's waking energy level?
○ low   ○ medium   ○ high

# of times roused from sleep last night?
○ 1   ○ 2   ○ 3+

Last night's reflux/GERD symptoms:

_____   _____

_____   _____

Bed raised?   ○ Y   ○ N   Wedged Pillows?   ○ Y   ○ N

Last meal time? _____   Approx bedtime? _____ am pm
(Remember to give yourself at least 2-3 hours after meals before lying down.)

End-of-day notes

Noticeable change in symptoms? _(Ex: "Throat discomfort has completely disappeared.")_

_____

_____

New terms to research   Books & websites with helpful info

_____   _____

_____   _____

Additional notes:

_____

_____

_____

Breakfast   Time: _____

List the foods you ate for breakfast.

_____   _____

_____   _____

_____   _____

Drink _____   **Drink** _____
  ○ room-temp ○ hot ○ cold   ○ room-temp ○ hot ○ cold

Comments:
_____

Physical symptoms after meal: ○ **low**   ○ **intense**   ○ **non-existent**
○ Belching   ○ Upper abdominal pain and discomfort
○ Nausea   ○ Difficulty or pain with swallowing
○ Stomach fullness or bloating   ○ Wheezing or dry cough

Other symptoms:
_____

Post-breakfast energy level: ○ low   ○ medium   ○ high

Lunch   Time: _____

List the foods you ate for lunch.

_____   _____

_____   _____

_____   _____

Drink _____   **Drink** _____
  ○ room-temp ○ hot ○ cold   ○ room-temp ○ hot ○ cold

Comments:
_____

Physical symptoms after meal: ○ **low**   ○ **intense**   ○ **non-existent**
○ Belching   ○ Upper abdominal pain and discomfort
○ Nausea   ○ Difficulty or pain with swallowing
○ Stomach fullness or bloating   ○ Wheezing or dry cough

Other symptoms:
_____

Post-lunch energy level: ○ low   ○ medium   ○ high

Dinner

Time: _____

List the foods you ate for dinner.

_____   _____

_____   _____

_____   _____

Drink _____   **Drink** _____
○ room-temp ○ hot ○ cold   ○ room-temp ○ hot ○ cold

Comments: _____

Physical symptoms after meal: ○ **low**   ○ **intense**   ○ **non-existent**
○ Belching   ○ Upper abdominal pain and discomfort
○ Nausea   ○ Difficulty or pain with swallowing
○ Stomach fullness or bloating   ○ Wheezing or dry cough

Other symptoms: _____

Post-dinner energy level: ○ low   ○ medium   ○ high

Snack

Time: _____

List the foods you ate as a snack.

_____   _____

Drink _____   ○ room-temp   ○ hot   ○ cold

Comments: _____

Post-snack energy level: ○ low   ○ medium   ○ high

Snack

Time: _____

List the foods you ate as a snack.

_____   _____

Drink _____   ○ room-temp   ○ hot   ○ cold

Comments: _____

Post-snack energy level: ○ low   ○ medium   ○ high

Medications & Supplements

Include prescription medication, over-the-counter medication & vitamin supplements.

_____   _____

_____   _____

_____   _____

_____   _____

_____   _____

Energy level | Restfulness

Today's waking energy level?
○ low   ○ medium   ○ high

# of times roused from sleep last night?
○ 1   ○ 2   ○ 3+

Last night's reflux/GERD symptoms:

_____   _____

_____   _____

Bed raised?   ○ Y   ○ N   Wedged Pillows?   ○ Y   ○ N

Last meal time? _____   Approx bedtime? _____ am   pm
(Remember to give yourself at least 2-3 hours after meals before lying down.)

End-of-day notes

Noticeable change in symptoms? *(Ex: "Throat discomfort has completely disappeared.")*

_____

_____

New terms to research   Books & websites with helpful info

_____   _____

_____   _____

Additional notes:

_____

_____

_____

Breakfast   Time: _____

List the foods you ate for breakfast.

_____   _____

_____   _____

_____   _____

Drink _____   **Drink** _____
○ room-temp   ○ hot   ○ cold   ○ room-temp   ○ hot   ○ cold

Comments: _____

Physical symptoms after meal: ○ **low**   ○ **intense**   ○ **non-existent**
○ Belching   ○ Upper abdominal pain and discomfort
○ Nausea   ○ Difficulty or pain with swallowing
○ Stomach fullness or bloating   ○ Wheezing or dry cough

Other symptoms: _____

Post-breakfast energy level: ○ low   ○ medium   ○ high

Lunch   Time: _____

List the foods you ate for lunch.

_____   _____

_____   _____

_____   _____

Drink _____   **Drink** _____
○ room-temp   ○ hot   ○ cold   ○ room-temp   ○ hot   ○ cold

Comments: _____

Physical symptoms after meal: ○ **low**   ○ **intense**   ○ **non-existent**
○ Belching   ○ Upper abdominal pain and discomfort
○ Nausea   ○ Difficulty or pain with swallowing
○ Stomach fullness or bloating   ○ Wheezing or dry cough

Other symptoms: _____

Post-lunch energy level: ○ low   ○ medium   ○ high

Dinner

Time: _____

List the foods you ate for dinner.

_____   _____

_____   _____

_____   _____

Drink _____   **Drink** _____
    ○ room-temp   ○ hot   ○ cold   ○ room-temp   ○ hot   ○ cold

Comments:

Physical symptoms after meal: ○ **low**   ○ **intense**   ○ **non-existent**
○ Belching   ○ Upper abdominal pain and discomfort
○ Nausea   ○ Difficulty or pain with swallowing
○ Stomach fullness or bloating   ○ Wheezing or dry cough

Other symptoms:

Post-dinner energy level: ○ low   ○ medium   ○ high

Snack

Time: _____

List the foods you ate as a snack.

_____   _____

Drink _____   ○ room-temp   ○ hot   ○ cold

Comments:

Post-snack energy level: ○ low   ○ medium   ○ high

Snack

Time: _____

List the foods you ate as a snack.

_____   _____

Drink _____   ○ room-temp   ○ hot   ○ cold

Comments:

Post-snack energy level: ○ low   ○ medium   ○ high

Medications & Supplements

Include prescription medication, over-the-counter medication & vitamin supplements.

_____   _____

_____   _____

_____   _____

_____   _____

_____   _____

Energy level | Restfulness

Today's waking energy level?
○ low   ○ medium   ○ high

# of times roused from sleep last night?
○ 1   ○ 2   ○ 3+

Last night's reflux/GERD symptoms:

_____   _____

_____   _____

Bed raised?   ○ Y   ○ N   Wedged Pillows?   ○ Y   ○ N

Last meal time? _____   Approx bedtime? _____   am   pm
(Remember to give yourself at least 2-3 hours after meals before lying down.)

End-of-day notes

Noticeable change in symptoms? *(Ex: "Throat discomfort has completely disappeared.")*

_____

_____

New terms to research   Books & websites with helpful info

_____   _____

_____   _____

Additional notes:

_____

_____

_____

Breakfast
Time: _____

List the foods you ate for breakfast.

_____   _____

_____   _____

_____   _____

Drink _____   **Drink** _____
  ○ room-temp   ○ hot   ○ cold   ○ room-temp   ○ hot   ○ cold

Comments: _____

Physical symptoms after meal: ○ **low**   ○ **intense**   ○ **non-existent**
○ Belching   ○ Upper abdominal pain and discomfort
○ Nausea   ○ Difficulty or pain with swallowing
○ Stomach fullness or bloating ○ Wheezing or dry cough

Other symptoms: _____

Post-breakfast energy level: ○ low   ○ medium   ○ high

Lunch
Time: _____

List the foods you ate for lunch.

_____   _____

_____   _____

_____   _____

Drink _____   **Drink** _____
  ○ room-temp   ○ hot   ○ cold   ○ room-temp   ○ hot   ○ cold

Comments: _____

Physical symptoms after meal: ○ **low**   ○ **intense**   ○ **non-existent**
○ Belching   ○ Upper abdominal pain and discomfort
○ Nausea   ○ Difficulty or pain with swallowing
○ Stomach fullness or bloating ○ Wheezing or dry cough

Other symptoms: _____

Post-lunch energy level: ○ low   ○ medium   ○ high

Dinner
Time: _____

List the foods you ate for dinner.

_____   _____

_____   _____

_____   _____

Drink _____   **Drink** _____
○ room-temp ○ hot ○ cold   ○ room-temp ○ hot ○ cold

Comments: _____

Physical symptoms after meal: ○ **low** ○ **intense** ○ **non-existent**
○ Belching   ○ Upper abdominal pain and discomfort
○ Nausea   ○ Difficulty or pain with swallowing
○ Stomach fullness or bloating   ○ Wheezing or dry cough

Other symptoms: _____

Post-dinner energy level: ○ low   ○ medium   ○ high

Snack
Time: _____

List the foods you ate as a snack.

_____   _____

Drink _____   ○ room-temp   ○ hot   ○ cold

Comments: _____

Post-snack energy level: ○ low   ○ medium   ○ high

Snack
Time: _____

List the foods you ate as a snack.

_____   _____

Drink _____   ○ room-temp   ○ hot   ○ cold

Comments: _____

Post-snack energy level: ○ low   ○ medium   ○ high

Medications & Supplements

Include prescription medication, over-the-counter medication & vitamin supplements.

_____   _____

_____   _____

_____   _____

_____   _____

_____

Energy level | Restfulness

Today's waking energy level?
○ low   ○ medium   ○ high

# of times roused from sleep last night?
○ 1   ○ 2   ○ 3+

Last night's reflux/GERD symptoms:

_____   _____

_____   _____

Bed raised?   ○ Y   ○ N   Wedged Pillows?   ○ Y   ○ N

Last meal time? _____   Approx bedtime? _____ am pm
(Remember to give yourself at least 2-3 hours after meals before lying down.)

End-of-day notes

Noticeable change in symptoms? _(Ex: "Throat discomfort has completely disappeared.")_

_____

_____

New terms to research   Books & websites with helpful info

_____   _____

_____   _____

Additional notes:

_____

_____

_____

_____

Breakfast   Time: _____

List the foods you ate for breakfast.

_____   _____

_____   _____

_____   _____

Drink _____   **Drink** _____
  ○ room-temp ○ hot ○ cold   ○ room-temp ○ hot ○ cold

Comments:

Physical symptoms after meal: ○ **low** ○ **intense** ○ **non-existent**
○ Belching   ○ Upper abdominal pain and discomfort
○ Nausea   ○ Difficulty or pain with swallowing
○ Stomach fullness or bloating   ○ Wheezing or dry cough

Other symptoms:

Post-breakfast energy level: ○ low ○ medium ○ high

Lunch   Time: _____

List the foods you ate for lunch.

_____   _____

_____   _____

_____   _____

Drink _____   **Drink** _____
  ○ room-temp ○ hot ○ cold   ○ room-temp ○ hot ○ cold

Comments:

Physical symptoms after meal: ○ **low** ○ **intense** ○ **non-existent**
○ Belching   ○ Upper abdominal pain and discomfort
○ Nausea   ○ Difficulty or pain with swallowing
○ Stomach fullness or bloating   ○ Wheezing or dry cough

Other symptoms:

Post-lunch energy level: ○ low ○ medium ○ high

Dinner

Time: _____

List the foods you ate for dinner.

_____   _____

_____   _____

_____   _____

Drink _____   **Drink** _____
○ room-temp   ○ hot   ○ cold   ○ room-temp   ○ hot   ○ cold

Comments: _____

Physical symptoms after meal: ○ **low**   ○ **intense**   ○ **non-existent**
○ Belching   ○ Upper abdominal pain and discomfort
○ Nausea   ○ Difficulty or pain with swallowing
○ Stomach fullness or bloating   ○ Wheezing or dry cough

Other symptoms: _____

Post-dinner energy level: ○ low   ○ medium   ○ high

Snack

Time: _____

List the foods you ate as a snack.

_____   _____

Drink _____   ○ room-temp   ○ hot   ○ cold

Comments: _____

Post-snack energy level: ○ low   ○ medium   ○ high

Snack

Time: _____

List the foods you ate as a snack.

_____   _____

Drink _____   ○ room-temp   ○ hot   ○ cold

Comments: _____

Post-snack energy level: ○ low   ○ medium   ○ high

Medications & Supplements

Include prescription medication, over-the-counter medication & vitamin supplements.

_____   _____

_____   _____

_____   _____

_____   _____

_____   _____

Energy level | Restfulness

Today's waking energy level?
○ low   ○ medium   ○ high

# of times roused from sleep last night?
○ 1   ○ 2   ○ 3+

Last night's reflux/GERD symptoms:

_____   _____

_____   _____

Bed raised?   ○ Y   ○ N   Wedged Pillows?   ○ Y   ○ N

Last meal time? _____   Approx bedtime? _____   am   pm
(Remember to give yourself at least 2-3 hours after meals before lying down.)

End-of-day notes

Noticeable change in symptoms? _(Ex: "Throat discomfort has completely disappeared.")_

_____

_____

New terms to research   Books & websites with helpful info

_____   _____

_____   _____

Additional notes:

_____

_____

_____

Breakfast

Time: _____

List the foods you ate for breakfast.

_____   _____

_____   _____

_____   _____

Drink _____   **Drink** _____
○ room-temp ○ hot ○ cold   ○ room-temp ○ hot ○ cold

Comments: _____

Physical symptoms after meal: ○ **low**   ○ **intense**   ○ **non-existent**
○ Belching   ○ Upper abdominal pain and discomfort
○ Nausea   ○ Difficulty or pain with swallowing
○ Stomach fullness or bloating   ○ Wheezing or dry cough

Other symptoms: _____

Post-breakfast energy level: ○ low   ○ medium   ○ high

Lunch

Time: _____

List the foods you ate for lunch.

_____   _____

_____   _____

_____   _____

Drink _____   **Drink** _____
○ room-temp ○ hot ○ cold   ○ room-temp ○ hot ○ cold

Comments: _____

Physical symptoms after meal: ○ **low**   ○ **intense**   ○ **non-existent**
○ Belching   ○ Upper abdominal pain and discomfort
○ Nausea   ○ Difficulty or pain with swallowing
○ Stomach fullness or bloating   ○ Wheezing or dry cough

Other symptoms: _____

Post-lunch energy level: ○ low   ○ medium   ○ high

Dinner

Time: _____

List the foods you ate for dinner.

_____   _____

_____   _____

_____   _____

Drink _____   **Drink** _____
  ○ room-temp ○ hot ○ cold   ○ room-temp ○ hot ○ cold

Comments: _____

Physical symptoms after meal: ○ **low**   ○ **intense**   ○ **non-existent**
  ○ Belching   ○ Upper abdominal pain and discomfort
  ○ Nausea   ○ Difficulty or pain with swallowing
  ○ Stomach fullness or bloating ○ Wheezing or dry cough

Other symptoms: _____

Post-dinner energy level: ○ low   ○ medium   ○ high

Snack

Time: _____

List the foods you ate as a snack.

_____   _____

Drink _____   ○ room-temp   ○ hot   ○ cold

Comments: _____

Post-snack energy level: ○ low   ○ medium   ○ high

Snack

Time: _____

List the foods you ate as a snack.

_____   _____

Drink _____   ○ room-temp   ○ hot   ○ cold

Comments: _____

Post-snack energy level: ○ low   ○ medium   ○ high

Medications & Supplements

Include prescription medication, over-the-counter medication & vitamin supplements.

_____   _____

_____   _____

_____   _____

_____   _____

_____   _____

Energy level | Restfulness

Today's waking energy level?
○ low   ○ medium   ○ high

# of times roused from sleep last night?
○ 1   ○ 2   ○ 3+

Last night's reflux/GERD symptoms:

_____   _____

_____   _____

Bed raised?   ○ Y   ○ N   Wedged Pillows?   ○ Y   ○ N

Last meal time? _____   Approx bedtime? _____ am pm
(Remember to give yourself at least 2-3 hours after meals before lying down.)

End-of-day notes

Noticeable change in symptoms? _(Ex: "Throat discomfort has completely disappeared.")_

_____

_____

New terms to research   Books & websites with helpful info

_____   _____

_____   _____

Additional notes:

_____

_____

_____

_____

Breakfast

Time: _____

List the foods you ate for breakfast.

_____   _____

_____   _____

_____   _____

Drink _____   **Drink** _____
○ room-temp ○ hot ○ cold   ○ room-temp ○ hot ○ cold

_____

Physical symptoms after meal: ○ **low**   ○ **intense**   ○ **non-existent**
○ Belching   ○ Upper abdominal pain and discomfort
○ Nausea   ○ Difficulty or pain with swallowing
○ Stomach fullness or bloating   ○ Wheezing or dry cough

Other symptoms: _____

Post-breakfast energy level: ○ low   ○ medium   ○ high

Lunch

Time: _____

List the foods you ate for lunch.

_____   _____

_____   _____

_____   _____

Drink _____   **Drink** _____
○ room-temp ○ hot ○ cold   ○ room-temp ○ hot ○ cold

Comments: _____

Physical symptoms after meal: ○ **low**   ○ **intense**   ○ **non-existent**
○ Belching   ○ Upper abdominal pain and discomfort
○ Nausea   ○ Difficulty or pain with swallowing
○ Stomach fullness or bloating   ○ Wheezing or dry cough

Other symptoms: _____

Post-lunch energy level: ○ low   ○ medium   ○ high

Dinner

Time: _____

List the foods you ate for dinner.

_____   _____

_____   _____

_____   _____

Drink _____   **Drink** _____
○ room-temp   ○ hot   ○ cold   ○ room-temp   ○ hot   ○ cold

Comments:

Physical symptoms after meal: ○ **low**   ○ **intense**   ○ **non-existent**
○ Belching   ○ Upper abdominal pain and discomfort
○ Nausea   ○ Difficulty or pain with swallowing
○ Stomach fullness or bloating   ○ Wheezing or dry cough

Other symptoms: _____

Post-dinner energy level: ○ low   ○ medium   ○ high

Snack

Time: _____

List the foods you ate as a snack.

_____   _____

Drink _____   ○ room-temp   ○ hot   ○ cold

Comments: _____

Post-snack energy level: ○ low   ○ medium   ○ high

Snack

Time: _____

List the foods you ate as a snack.

_____   _____

Drink _____   ○ room-temp   ○ hot   ○ cold

Comments: _____

Post-snack energy level: ○ low   ○ medium   ○ high

Medications & Supplements

Include prescription medication, over-the-counter medication & vitamin supplements.

_____   _____

_____   _____

_____   _____

_____   _____

_____   _____

Energy level | Restfulness

Today's waking energy level?
○ low   ○ medium   ○ high

# of times roused from sleep last night?
○ 1   ○ 2   ○ 3+

Last night's reflux/GERD symptoms:

_____   _____

_____   _____

Bed raised?   ○ Y   ○ N   Wedged Pillows?   ○ Y   ○ N

Last meal time? _____   Approx bedtime? _____ am pm
(Remember to give yourself at least 2-3 hours after meals before lying down.)

End-of-day notes

Noticeable change in symptoms? *(Ex: "Throat discomfort has completely disappeared.")*

_____

_____

New terms to research   Books & websites with helpful info

_____   _____

_____   _____

Additional notes:

_____

_____

_____

_____

Breakfast   Time: _____

List the foods you ate for breakfast.

_____   _____

_____   _____

_____   _____

Drink _____   **Drink** _____
  ○ room-temp   ○ hot   ○ cold   ○ room-temp   ○ hot   ○ cold

Comments: _____

Physical symptoms after meal: ○ **low**   ○ **intense**   ○ **non-existent**
○ Belching   ○ Upper abdominal pain and discomfort
○ Nausea   ○ Difficulty or pain with swallowing
○ Stomach fullness or bloating   ○ Wheezing or dry cough

Other symptoms: _____

Post-breakfast energy level: ○ low   ○ medium   ○ high

Lunch   Time: _____

List the foods you ate for lunch.

_____   _____

_____   _____

_____   _____

Drink _____   **Drink** _____
  ○ room-temp   ○ hot   ○ cold   ○ room-temp   ○ hot   ○ cold

Comments: _____

Physical symptoms after meal: ○ **low**   ○ **intense**   ○ **non-existent**
○ Belching   ○ Upper abdominal pain and discomfort
○ Nausea   ○ Difficulty or pain with swallowing
○ Stomach fullness or bloating   ○ Wheezing or dry cough

Other symptoms: _____

Post-lunch energy level: ○ low   ○ medium   ○ high

Dinner

Time: _____

List the foods you ate for dinner.

_____   _____

_____   _____

_____   _____

Drink _____   **Drink** _____
○ room-temp ○ hot ○ cold   ○ room-temp ○ hot ○ cold

Comments: _____

Physical symptoms after meal: ○ **low** ○ **intense** ○ **non-existent**
○ Belching   ○ Upper abdominal pain and discomfort
○ Nausea   ○ Difficulty or pain with swallowing
○ Stomach fullness or bloating   ○ Wheezing or dry cough

Other symptoms: _____

Post-dinner energy level: ○ low ○ medium ○ high

Snack

Time: _____

List the foods you ate as a snack.

_____   _____

Drink _____ ○ room-temp ○ hot ○ cold

Comments: _____

Post-snack energy level: ○ low ○ medium ○ high

Snack

Time: _____

List the foods you ate as a snack.

_____   _____

Drink _____ ○ room-temp ○ hot ○ cold

Comments: _____

Post-snack energy level: ○ low ○ medium ○ high

Medications & Supplements

Include prescription medication, over-the-counter medication & vitamin supplements.

_____   _____

_____   _____

_____   _____

_____   _____

_____   _____

Energy level | Restfulness

Today's waking energy level?
○ low   ○ medium   ○ high

# of times roused from sleep last night?
○ 1   ○ 2   ○ 3+

Last night's reflux/GERD symptoms:

_____   _____

_____   _____

Bed raised?   ○ Y   ○ N   Wedged Pillows?   ○ Y   ○ N

Last meal time? _____   Approx bedtime? _____   am   pm

(Remember to give yourself at least 2-3 hours after meals before lying down.)

End-of-day notes

Noticeable change in symptoms? _(Ex: "Throat discomfort has completely disappeared.")_

_____

_____

New terms to research   Books & websites with helpful info

_____   _____

_____   _____

Additional notes:

_____

_____

_____

_____

Breakfast

Time: _____

List the foods you ate for breakfast.

_____   _____

_____   _____

_____   _____

Drink _____   **Drink** _____
  ○ room-temp ○ hot ○ cold   ○ room-temp ○ hot ○ cold

Comments: _____

Physical symptoms after meal: ○ **low** ○ **intense** ○ **non-existent**
○ Belching   ○ Upper abdominal pain and discomfort
○ Nausea   ○ Difficulty or pain with swallowing
○ Stomach fullness or bloating   ○ Wheezing or dry cough

Other symptoms: _____

Post-breakfast energy level: ○ low ○ medium ○ high

Lunch

Time: _____

List the foods you ate for lunch.

_____   _____

_____   _____

_____   _____

Drink _____   **Drink** _____
  ○ room-temp ○ hot ○ cold   ○ room-temp ○ hot ○ cold

Comments: _____

Physical symptoms after meal: ○ **low** ○ **intense** ○ **non-existent**
○ Belching   ○ Upper abdominal pain and discomfort
○ Nausea   ○ Difficulty or pain with swallowing
○ Stomach fullness or bloating   ○ Wheezing or dry cough

Other symptoms: _____

Post-lunch energy level: ○ low ○ medium ○ high

Dinner   Time: _____

List the foods you ate for dinner.

_____   _____

_____   _____

_____   _____

Drink _____   **Drink** _____
○ room-temp ○ hot ○ cold   ○ room-temp ○ hot ○ cold

Comments:
_____

Physical symptoms after meal: ○ **low**   ○ **intense**   ○ **non-existent**
○ Belching   ○ Upper abdominal pain and discomfort
○ Nausea   ○ Difficulty or pain with swallowing
○ Stomach fullness or bloating ○ Wheezing or dry cough

Other symptoms: _____

Post-dinner energy level: ○ low   ○ medium   ○ high

Snack   Time: _____

List the foods you ate as a snack.

_____   _____

Drink _____   ○ room-temp   ○ hot   ○ cold

Comments: _____

Post-snack energy level: ○ low   ○ medium   ○ high

Snack   Time: _____

List the foods you ate as a snack.

_____   _____

Drink _____   ○ room-temp   ○ hot   ○ cold

Comments: _____

Post-snack energy level: ○ low   ○ medium   ○ high

Medications & Supplements

Include prescription medication, over-the-counter medication & vitamin supplements.

_____   _____

_____   _____

_____   _____

_____   _____

_____

Energy level | Restfulness

Today's waking energy level?
○ low   ○ medium   ○ high

# of times roused from sleep last night?
○ 1   ○ 2   ○ 3+

Last night's reflux/GERD symptoms:

_____   _____

_____   _____

Bed raised?   ○ Y   ○ N   Wedged Pillows?   ○ Y   ○ N

Last meal time? _____   Approx bedtime? _____ am pm
(Remember to give yourself at least 2-3 hours after meals before lying down.)

End-of-day notes

Noticeable change in symptoms? *(Ex: "Throat discomfort has completely disappeared.")*

_____

_____

New terms to research   Books & websites with helpful info

_____   _____

_____   _____

Additional notes:

_____

_____

_____

Breakfast   Time: _____

List the foods you ate for breakfast.

_____   _____

_____   _____

_____   _____

Drink _____   **Drink** _____
  ○ room-temp ○ hot ○ cold   ○ room-temp ○ hot ○ cold

Comments: _____

Physical symptoms after meal: ○ **low**   ○ **intense**   ○ **non-existent**
○ Belching   ○ Upper abdominal pain and discomfort
○ Nausea   ○ Difficulty or pain with swallowing
○ Stomach fullness or bloating   ○ Wheezing or dry cough

Other symptoms: _____

Post-breakfast energy level: ○ low   ○ medium   ○ high

Lunch   Time: _____

List the foods you ate for lunch.

_____   _____

_____   _____

_____   _____

Drink _____   **Drink** _____
  ○ room-temp ○ hot ○ cold   ○ room-temp ○ hot ○ cold

Comments: _____

Physical symptoms after meal: ○ **low**   ○ **intense**   ○ **non-existent**
○ Belching   ○ Upper abdominal pain and discomfort
○ Nausea   ○ Difficulty or pain with swallowing
○ Stomach fullness or bloating   ○ Wheezing or dry cough

Other symptoms: _____

Post-lunch energy level: ○ low   ○ medium   ○ high

Dinner
Time: _____

List the foods you ate for dinner.

_____   _____

_____   _____

_____   _____

Drink _____   **Drink** _____
○ room-temp   ○ hot   ○ cold   ○ room-temp   ○ hot   ○ cold

Comments: _____

Physical symptoms after meal: ○ **low**   ○ **intense**   ○ **non-existent**
○ Belching   ○ Upper abdominal pain and discomfort
○ Nausea   ○ Difficulty or pain with swallowing
○ Stomach fullness or bloating   ○ Wheezing or dry cough

Other symptoms: _____

Post-dinner energy level: ○ low   ○ medium   ○ high

Snack
Time: _____

List the foods you ate as a snack.

_____   _____

Drink _____   ○ room-temp   ○ hot   ○ cold

Comments: _____

Post-snack energy level: ○ low   ○ medium   ○ high

Snack
Time: _____

List the foods you ate as a snack.

_____   _____

Drink _____   ○ room-temp   ○ hot   ○ cold

Comments: _____

Post-snack energy level: ○ low   ○ medium   ○ high

Medications & Supplements

Include prescription medication, over-the-counter medication & vitamin supplements.

_____   _____

_____   _____

_____   _____

_____   _____

_____   _____

Energy level | Restfulness

Today's waking energy level?
○ low   ○ medium   ○ high

# of times roused from sleep last night?
○ 1   ○ 2   ○ 3+

Last night's reflux/GERD symptoms:

_____   _____

_____   _____

Bed raised?   ○ Y   ○ N   Wedged Pillows?   ○ Y   ○ N

Last meal time? _____   Approx bedtime? _____   am   pm

(Remember to give yourself at least 2-3 hours after meals before lying down.)

End-of-day notes

Noticeable change in symptoms? _(Ex: "Throat discomfort has completely disappeared.")_

_____

_____

New terms to research   Books & websites with helpful info

_____   _____

_____   _____

Additional notes:

_____

_____

_____

79241720R00102

Made in the USA
Middletown, DE
08 July 2018